Clinical Procedures in Primary Eye Care

Clinical Procedures in Primary Eye Care

Editor

David B. Elliott BSc PhD MCOptom FAAO

*Clinic Director, Senior Lecturer, Department of Optometry,
University of Bradford, UK*

John Flanagan BSc PhD FCOptom FAAO
*Professor of Optometry, School of Optometry, University of Waterloo, Professor of
Ophthalmology, Department of Ophthalmology, University of Toronto, Canada, and Visiting
Professor, Department of Optometry, School of Biomedical Sciences, University of Ulster,
Coleraine, N. Ireland*

Patricia Hrynchak OD FAAO
*Assistant Clinic Director and Head of Primary Care Clinic, Lecturer, School of Optometry,
University of Waterloo, Canada*

Mark Hurst BSc PhD FCOptom FAAO
Head of Diabetic Clinic, Lecturer, Department of Optometry, University of Bradford, UK

C. Lisa Prokopich BSc OD FAAO
*Head of Ocular Health and Hospital Clinics, Lecturer, School of Optometry, University of
Waterloo, Canada*

Barry Winn BSc PhD MCOptom
*Professor of Optometry, Head of Department, Department of Optometry, University of Bradford,
UK*

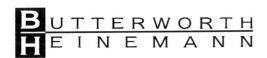

Butterworth-Heinemann Ltd
Linacre House, Jordan Hill, Oxford OX2 8DP
A division of Reed Educational and Professional Publishing Ltd

 A member of the Reed Elsevier plc group

OXFORD   BOSTON   JOHANNESBURG
MELBOURNE   NEW DELHI   SINGAPORE

First published 1997

British Library Cataloguing in Publication Data

Clinical procedures in primary eye care
  1. Eye – Examination 2 Eye – Diseases – Diagnosis
  I. Elliott, David B.
  617. 7'15

  ISBN 0 7506 3213 5

Library of Congress Cataloguing in Publication Data

Clinical procedures in primary eye care/editor, David B. Elliott:
  John Flanagan ... [et al.].
    p.   cm.
  Includes bibliographical references and index
  ISBN 0 7506 3213 5
  1. Optometry – Handbooks, manuals, etc.   I. Elliott, David B.
  II. Flanagan, John, Ph.D.
  [DNLM: 1. Vision Disorders – diagnosis – handbooks. 2. Vision Tests –
  handbooks 3. Ocular Motility Disorders – diagnosis – handbooks. 4. Vision
  Disorders – therapy – handbooks.   5. Optometry – methods – handbooks.
  WW 39 C641 1997]
  RE952 9 C56 1997
  617. dc21   97-25703
                                                                      CIP

Typeset by Keyword Typesetting Services Ltd., Wallington, Surrey
Printed and bound in Great Britain by Bath Press Plc, Avon.

Contents

Preface

This manual is a guideline to clinical procedures in primary eye care, and was written primarily as a teaching aid for undergraduate optometry students. Although it is not intended to be inclusive of all techniques that can be performed in optometric practice, the majority of the most popular procedures in the UK are covered. The manual may also be of interest to practitioners as it includes several diagnostic and treatment procedures which are relatively new to UK optometry and with which they may be unfamiliar, such as binocular indirect ophthalmoscopy and punctal plug insertion. For the majority of functions or states which can be tested in an eye examination, some background information is provided, then a recommended test is indicated and described in detail. For each recommended test, the following aspects are discussed: the rationale behind choosing the test recommended; the measurement procedure; how to record the results of the test; how to interpret the results; a list of errors most commonly made by students (with an attempt to put the most common first) and some key references.

The manual is divided into six chapters and the full contents can be seen by looking at the Contents page. In summary, Chapter 1 is an introduction and includes a discussion of what constitutes an optometric examination and the importance of, and how to perform, a case history. Chapter 2 discusses preliminary tests which are all those procedures generally performed prior to refraction such as visual acuity, colour vision and inter-pupillary distance measurement. Chapter 3 discusses refraction and includes objective and subjective refraction and near addition assessment. Chapter 4 discusses post-refractive binocular vision testing and includes the assessment of accommodation, fixation disparity, and stereopsis amongst many others. Some procedures can be performed both before and after refraction, such as visual acuity, cover test and fixation disparity. These are described in detail only in the preliminary or post-refractive testing sections. Chapter 5 discusses all aspects of the assessment of ocular health. Practitioners may be interested in sections on automated visual field assessment, gonioscopy, fundus biomicroscopy, binocular indirect ophthalmoscopy and the Jones' tests for assessment of patency of the lacrimal drainage system. Chapter 6 deals with treatment options, and covers the full range of treatment regimes from spectacle prescribing to patient counselling to prophylactic and therapeutic drugs, foreign body removal and lacrimal plugs.

Comments and suggestions for future editions

For each recommended procedure, the rationale for its inclusion is given and where appropriate it is compared to any alternatives. We have also tried to include various alternative procedures which are commonly used (with their advantages and disadvantages). However, no doubt tests and test methodologies have been included which may reflect our biases due to particular training, research and clinical experience. There may be errors and omissions also. Therefore we welcome any comments and suggestions which would improve any further editions of this manual. Please write to the editor, Dr David Elliott, at the Department of Optometry, University of Bradford, Bradford BD7 1DP, UK.

Information relevant to students

The order of the test procedures is loosely based on their order in an eye examination. It is not based on the order the procedures will be taught in clinical optometry courses. In these courses, procedures which require considerable practice, such as retinoscopy, ophthalmoscopy and subjective refraction, tend to be taught first and the eye examination is built up from this base. In addition, some aspects of the eye examination such as the problem-oriented approach can be taught only after students have a considerable knowledge base from which to work, and therefore appear later in the curriculum.

The recommendations in this manual are just that and not hard and fast rules. There are many approaches to conducting an eye examination and different ways to perform various tests or procedures properly. Any methods or tests which are not in this manual are not in any way 'wrong'. Indeed, the tests and test methodologies included no doubt reflect biases due to particular training, research and clinical experience. In particular, in university primary care clinics it is the supervising clinician's decision as to which techniques or tests should be used in an eye examination. They are taking legal responsibility for the examination. If they indicate that a particular test needs to be used, use it!

Acknowledgements

The inspiration behind this manual was *Clinical Procedures in Optometry* (P. Hrynchak, ed.), University of Waterloo Press, on which this manual is based. Some sections in the manual have been adapted from that textbook.

We wish to thank Anne Weber (University of Waterloo) for several of the figures; Claire Green, Jim Gilchrist, Stewart Mitchell, Tony Shakespeare, Shahina Pardhan and Henry Burek (University of Bradford) for valuable comments, and the students of the Department of Optometry at Bradford for spotting the mistakes in an earlier version of the manual.

Finally we wish to especially thank our families and partners for their support and their understanding of the time commitment required to produce this manual: Mary Elliott, Kathy Dumbleton, Walter Mittelstaedt, Val Hurst, Randy Roenspiess and Beth Winn.

1
Introduction

What constitutes an optometric examination?

There are various definitions of what constitutes an optometric examination. There is a legal definition and a College of Optometrists definition. The style of examination could be determined by the assessment of a series of tests (database style examination), by the assessment of several systems (systems approach) and/or using the problem-oriented approach.

Legal definition

The legal requirements of an optometric examination (occasionally still known under the outdated title of a 'sight test') in the UK are determined by the Optician's Act 1989 and several following Statutory Instruments (SIs). The pertinent points are that the optometric examination must:

1. Detect ocular abnormality.
2. Specify functional corrections for eye defects.

College of Optometrists' guidelines

The College of Optometrists provides guidelines for what constitutes an eye examination in its code of ethics and guidelines for professional conduct (latest revision March 1991). If the General Optical Council were to investigate an optometrist in a disciplinary matter *re* the extent of his or her examination, they have indicated that they would interpret these guidelines as the 'peer view' examination. Point 1.5.3 of these guidelines indicates that:

1. In every case the eye examination must be carried out thoroughly in relation to the particular needs of each patient.
2. The purpose of the eye examination is to identify the patient's precise needs for vision care, by:
   (a) Detecting ocular abnormality.
   (b) Prescribing functional corrections for defects of sight.

(c) Suggesting or providing remedial visual training where appropriate.

(d) Providing advice to the patient on all aspects of visual efficiency.

3. The eye examination as practitioners have been trained to carry it out includes the following:

(a) Complete assessment of history and symptoms.
(b) Assessment of the patient's visual needs and visual environments.
(c) Aided and/or unaided vision of each eye (aided vision must be accompanied by the specific prescription used).
(d) Ocular motility, convergence, pupil reflexes.
(e) Screening for visual field defects.
(f) Internal and external examination of the eyes.
(g) Objective refractive findings.
(h) Monocular distance subjective findings to establish visual acuity of each eye.
(i) Binocular balancing and binocular visual acuity if appropriate
(j) Distance oculo-motor assessment.
(k) Assessment of accommodation (distance Rx *in situ*) to assess any additions to the distance prescription, if required.
(l) Near oculo-motor assessment.
(m) Any other relevant tests necessary.
(n) Final determination of correction needed.

4. Findings should be recorded. If findings are not recorded, it cannot be assumed that the relevant test has been carried out.
5. It is for each practitioner to exercise his or her professional judgement as to precisely which tests are relevant to the interests of individual patients (see 3(m) above). It should be borne in mind that as the public becomes better informed as to the full extent of an eye examination, patients will expect to be satisfied that all the tests appropriate to their needs have been carried out. It is increasingly necessary to explain what is happening and why.

These guidelines could therefore be interpreted in two ways. Either every eye examination must include all the procedures listed in 3 (above), or it is for each practitioner to exercise his or her professional judgement as to precisely which tests are relevant to the interests of individual patients.

Given that it would be impossible to complete all the indicated procedures when examining some patients, such as young children or monocular patients, the second interpretation seems more appropriate, and this is the usual interpretation made (e.g. Taylor and Austen, 1992). Therefore the minimum requirements remain those indicated by the legal definition, with perhaps the extra requirement that optometrists should suggest or provide remedial visual training where appropriate.

Database style examination

A database-oriented examination style means using essentially the same set of clinical procedures in every examination. A large 'complete' database of information is collected to ensure that most patients' problems can be addressed using the information provided. This is the style of examination that will be used by students, particularly in the first years of learning. Practising the various clinical techniques is required, so that students are technically competent at performing each technique. Technical competence should be the aim for students after the first year's teaching. A much greater task is gaining clinical competence. What do all the tests mean and how do they interact? How do you use test results to solve the patient's problems?, etc. etc. Only once a student/practitioner has gained a high level of clinical competence should the database style of examination be abandoned and a problem-oriented examination used.

Although the database examination style is ideal for students, it is not for practitioners. If patients require additional testing, because of the inflexibility of the approach, practitioners either perform the tests at the end of the examination (which can lead to them being late for subsequent examinations) or another appointment is made at a later date. This has the disadvantage that it can bias against performing the extra tests, particularly as there is generally no extra income derived from performing these extra procedures. Practitioners may convince themselves that there is no real need for the additional procedures, may re-book the patient for another examination in 6 months' time, or may refer the patients to their general practitioner for further examination. At its worst, this style of examination could be said to provide some test data which are not used and of little value, and provides a bias against performing additional procedures which may be of real benefit.

Systems examination

A systems examination style includes an assessment of the motor, refractive and sensory systems and an assessment of the structures responsible for their function (ocular health assessment). The optometric examination is defined not by the specifics of tests used but, more importantly, by the visual functions and/or structures that these tests examine. This approach is much more flexible as it does not demand that a certain collection of tests be used. Using a 'collection of tests' style examination, the test list needs to be continually updated as technological and research advances change the examination requirements. For example, can contemporary autorefractors be used instead of static retinoscopy? Given the research evidence that tonometry screening in glaucoma is inefficient on its own, should this procedure be augmented or replaced by visual field screening? A systems examination style is much more adaptable as this updating is not required. In such an examination style, a minimum data base has been gathered when each system has been tested. In summary, think in terms of assessing systems and not of using individual tests (Table 1.1).

Problem-oriented examination

The problem-oriented examination is built upon a systems examination approach. In addition, it aligns the examination around the expressed problems of the patient. As it is based on the systems approach, this is not exclusive. For example, it is not sufficient to perform only case history, visual acuity and refraction on a patient who complains of blurred distance vision. There are many obvious reasons why such an approach is flawed, including the fact that important sight-threatening conditions can be symptomless and should be detected by the optometrist.

By design, a database-oriented examination often collects a lot of data that do not address the patient's problem(s). The expanding scope of optometric practice continues to add extra procedures to the traditional basic optometric operations. Providing comprehensive contemporary optometric care that includes these new techniques, as well as the old ones, requires selective streamlining of the examination routine. The problem-solving approach is one way to rationalise this streamlining of the examination without compromising the quality of patient care. This involves measuring routinely only those tests which are considered essential for performing a competent, legal examination. Additional tests to this reduced database are used when signs and symptoms suggest, i.e. the procedures used in every examination are likely to be different and are guided by the patient's problems. This style of examination does use a reduced database, and various tests which are measured routinely in a database style of examination are not measured routinely in a problem-oriented approach.

Several questions should be considered when deciding which tests should be part of an optometric examination:

1. Do I really understand what the tests are measuring, and do they provide significant decision-making information?
2. Am I using the minimum amount of procedures to yield the maximum amount of information?

Table 1.1 Classification of clinical tests into one of the four oculo-visual systems

Refractive	Sensory	Motor	Ocular health
Case history	Case history	Case history	Case history
Keratometry	Visual acuity	Accommodation	Ophthalmoscopy
Retinoscopy	Stereoacuity	Phorias	Biomicroscopy
Autorefraction	Contrast sensitivity	Fusion limits	Tonometry
Subjective	Visual fields	Pursuits	Gonioscopy
	Colour vision	Saccades	Pupil responses
	Suppression	Pupil responses	

To perform a problem-oriented examination, the case history is critical as it guides the whole examination. From the information gained in the case history, the clinician should attempt to deduce a list of tentative diagnoses. For example, a symptom of blurred vision in a teenager could suggest the following tentative diagnoses (in order of likelihood): myopia, pseudomyopia, malingering, ocular hysteria, diabetes mellitus. Throughout the examination the clinician must decide whether additional tests are required to help in differential diagnosis. Although the problem-oriented examination requires a minimal database as required for legal reasons and to ensure that each system is assessed, this is obviously not its major characteristic. Rather, it is distinguished by its variability. For example, if a 12-year-old patient complains of frontal headaches and eyestrain when reading, the most likely tentative diagnoses are uncorrected hypermetropia or a near heterophoria problem. Depending on results from other tests, tests used may include measuring fusional reserves, ratio of accommodative convergence to accommodation (AC/A ratio), fixation disparity and cycloplegic refraction. If a 30-year-old patient is complaining of sudden painless vision loss in one eye (> 24 hours), the most likely tentative diagnoses would include a unilateral change in refractive error (i.e. suddenly noticed rather than sudden onset), optic neuritis and idiopathic central serous choroidopathy. None of the additional tests used in the previous example would be used. Instead, fundus biomicroscopy, photostress recovery time, Amsler grid, red cap and contrast sensitivity testing may be used. When using this style of examination, you must also be aware that any new or changed prescription should not produce symptoms. For example, the effect of a new myopic Rx on an esophoria should be determined.

Disadvantages of the problem-oriented examination include its dependence on the patient's symptoms. Obviously if a case history is not possible for any reason, a problem-oriented approach cannot be used and a database style of examination is necessary. Similarly, some patients are not articulate enough to provide a good case history and a database style of examination should again be used. Some patients may not disclose all their symptoms, since they might believe that their headaches are not associated with their vision or their eyes, or that their slightly blurred vision, headaches or diplopia are normal consequences of ageing. Because of a reduced database, the cause of these non-revealed symptoms may be missed in a problem-oriented examination. To perform a problem-oriented examination, a competent grasp of the information provided in the case history and how it relates to various ocular abnormalities is needed, plus a knowledge of which tests are required to perform the huge variety of differential diagnoses.

Combination approach

It can be useful to gain a complete database of information during an initial examination of a patient, and then use a problem-oriented approach during subsequent examinations. This necessitates different appointment slots for first time and subsequent examinations, with the first time appointment slot being longer than for subsequent visits. This type of combination approach appears to glean the best elements of the two examination styles.

Use of clinical assistants and their effect on the optometric examination

Increasingly, clinical assistants are being used to perform routinely various automated or simple tests. The rationale behind this approach is twofold:

1. These procedures generally become more routinely performed thereby improving patient quality of care.
2. The clinical assistant's time is less expensive than an optometrist's and by having them routinely perform certain tests that the optometrist would previously have performed, some of the optometrist's time is freed up. The optometrist can use this extra time to perform some of the extra procedures which are being added to the traditional basic optometric operations, such as binocular indirect ophthalmoscopy and fundus biomicroscopy. In addition, the time spent with the optometrist may be reduced, allowing him or her to examine more patients per day without compromising the quality of patient care.

What procedures and tests can a clinical assistant perform? After a period of training, they should be able to perform competently any automated procedure, such as automated visual fields and focimetry, autorefraction and non-contact tonometry. In addition, other simple tests could be performed, such as colour vision and stereopsis screening, interpupillary distance measurement and perhaps even Maddox wing assessment with the patient's own spectacles. It is not possible for a clinical assistant to complete the full case history, since history taking continues throughout the examination. However, assistants could record a baseline history which could be reviewed and augmented by the optometrist. I personally do not favour this approach as it provides less likelihood of a good rapport being established between patient and clinician, which seems vital for an optimal examination result. Clinical assistants could also measure visual acuity with the patient's spectacles. However, important information can be obtained during visual acuity measurement in addition to the acuity score and, as an important part of the subjective refraction is to compare the final visual acuity (which the optometrist measures) with the habitual acuity, it appears best to have both measurements made by the optometrist.

The vital importance of good training and continuing education of clinical assistants should be obvious.

Amos, J.F. (1987). The problem-solving approach to patient care. In *Diagnosis and Management in Vision Care* (J.F. Amos, ed.) Butterworth–Heinemann, Oxford, UK

Elliott, D.B. (1997). The problem-oriented examination's case history. In *The Ocular Examination: Measurements and Findings* (K. Zadnik, ed.) W.B. Saunders, London, UK

Taylor, S.P. and Austen, D.P. (1992). *Law and Management in Optometric Practice*. Butterworth–Heinemann, Oxford, UK

Record forms

It is essential that all test results (including the 'results' from case history) are recorded. If they are not recorded, they were not performed. In each of the following sections, a subsection on recording is included.

Many record forms are produced with various designated areas for certain test results which are commonly performed. This is an attempt to save time as you do not have to write down the test or procedure used, but merely the result. Many different record cards will be encountered by a locum optometrist, and there is no standard at present. The College of Optometrists is presently working on producing recommended record cards for the various types of optometric examination (principally primary care and contact lenses). As an example, the record form used at the University of Bradford is shown in Figure 1.1. It has been designed for student use and for a database style of examination and is not recommended for practitioners.

Problem-oriented record form

The problem-oriented examination uses the acronym SOAP for its record format. SOAP stands for Subjective, Objective, Assessment, Plan. The record card itself is a plain white sheet; this reflects the fact that this style of examination is distinguished by its variability, so there is little point in making boxes for individual tests. The subjective information is that obtained from the case history and the objective information comprises the various test results obtained during the examination. The assessment and plan refer to the problem–plan list which is described in detail in a later section.

Test order

Table 1.2 provides a suggested order of testing for performing an efficient optometric examination. The exact testing to be performed will depend on

	UNIVERSITY OF BRADFORD	EYE EXAMINATION RECORD CARD

Px ID

FIRST NAME :   AGE :   DATE :

SURNAME: DOB:

ADDRESS :   TEL NO :

CASE HISTORY

CC :

Present Rx   DBC   /

	SPH	CYL	AXIS	Δ	BC
R					
L					
	ADD	SEG STYLE	SEG HT	☐ CR39 ☐ GLASS ☐ OTHER	TINT

Sports/hobbies :
Driver? :

OH :

GH :   MEDS :   ALLERGIES :

FOH :   LEE :

FMH :   LME :

GP:

PRELIMINARY TESTING

VISION (DV) : (R)   (L)   (B)   VISION (NV @   cms) : (R)   (L)   (B)

VA (DV) : (R)   (L)   (B)   VA (NV @   cms) : (R)   (L)   (B)

☐ SPECTACLES ☐ CONTACT LENSES

COVER TEST
          Distance   Near   NPC _____ cms   MOTILITY

Unaided   JUMP C

Aided   CONFRONTATION FIELDS

          PD _____ / _____

REFRACTION

OBJECTIVE REFRACTION

(R)   VA   (L)   VA

☐ RETINOSCOPY ☐ AUTOREFRACTOR ☐ OTHER

SUBJECTIVE REFRACTION   Vertex distance   mm

(R)   VA   (L)   VA

☐ HUMPHRISS ☐ PRISM DISS ☐ TIB ☐ POLARISATION ☐ MONOCULAR ☐ OTHER

BINOCULAR ADD : _____   READING ADD @ _____ cms

TENTATIVE READING ADD   ☐ AGE   (R)   N____   (L)   N____
                          ☐ Rx
(R)   (L)   ☐ X-CYL   (B)   Range from _____ to _____ cms
                          ☐ AMPS

BINOCULAR   VISION

AMPLITUDE OF ACCOMMODATION   STEREOPSIS

(R)   (L)   (B)

☐ PUSH-UP ☐ TROMBONE ☐ SHEARDS   ☐ TNO ☐ TITMUS ☐ FRISBY ☐ RANDOT ☐ LANG

MUSCLE BALANCE   FIXATION DISPARITY
          Distance   Near   Distance   Near
H   H

V   V

☐ COVER TEST ☐ COVER TEST/PRISMS ☐ MADDOX ☐ OTHER   ☐ MALLETT ☐ FREEMAN ☐ OTHER

Figure 1.1(a)

| OCULAR HEALTH | TONOMETRY   Time:

 (R)   (L)

 □ GOLDMAN/PERKINS   □ NCT   □ PULSAIR   □ OTHER | □ YES
 SENSITIVITY TO Dx DRUGS
        □ NO
 ANTERIOR ANGLE   □ VAN HERICK   □ RATIO   □ PENLIGHT
 (R)   T.   N.   (L)   T.   N. |

| | ANTERIOR SEGMENT   □ SLIT-LAMP   □ DIRECT
                  □ OTHER   □ LOUPE
           (R)   (L)
 Lids & margins
 Conjunctiva
 Cornea
 Sclera
 Ant. Chamber
 Iris
 Pupil
 Lens

 Pupil reflexes :

 Marcus-Gunn : | POSTERIOR SEGMENT   □ BIO   □ BIOMICROSCOPE
                        □ MIO
 Mydriatic _____   □ DIRECT   □ PHOTO
 Post-mydriatic IOP _____
              (R)   (L)
 Vitreous
 Disc
 C/D ratios (H)
              (V)
 Retinal vessels
 A/V ratios
 Posterior pole
 Macula
 Periphery |

SUPPLEMENTARY TESTING

SUPPLEMENTARY TESTING (e.g. Visual fields, cycloplegic refraction, colour vision, contrast sensitivity)

SUMMARY

#	PROBLEM	#	PLAN
--	-------------------------------	--	-------------------------------
--	-------------------------------	--	-------------------------------
--	-------------------------------	--	-------------------------------
--	-------------------------------	--	-------------------------------
--	-------------------------------	--	-------------------------------
--	-------------------------------	--	-------------------------------
--	-------------------------------	--	-------------------------------
--	-------------------------------	--	-------------------------------
--	-------------------------------	--	-------------------------------
--	-------------------------------	--	-------------------------------
--	-------------------------------	--	-------------------------------
--	-------------------------------	--	-------------------------------
--	-------------------------------	--	-------------------------------

PRESCRIPTION

	SPH	CYL	AXIS	Δ	Vertex dist.	NV ADD	DBC	Student Clinican's Name:
R								
L							/	Student's Signature:

OTHER INFORMATION (E.G. INTERMEDIATE ADD):   Supervising Clinician's Signature:

Figure 1.1(a) and (b) (cont.) The record form used in primary care clinics at the University of Bradford. (Reprinted with permission.)

9

Table 1.2 Suggested order for performing various procedures in an optometric examination

Patient identifying information
Case history
Preliminary tests
   Focimetry
   Vision
      Distance
      Near
   Unaided cover test (distance and/or near)
   Aided visual acuity
      Distance
      Near
   Aided cover test (distance and/or near)
   Near point of convergence
   Motility
Refraction
   Interpupillary distance
   Retinoscopy
   Monocular subjective refraction
   Balanced subjective refraction or binocular refraction
Binocular vision tests
   Distance cover test (or alternative)
   Amplitude of accommodation
   Reading add determination – if indicated
   Near cover test (or alternative)
   Fixation disparity
   Stereoacuity
Ocular Health Assessment
   Pupil reflexes
   Direct ophthalmoscopy (if not performing indirect ophthalmoscopy)
   Anterior angle assessment
   Slit lamp examination
   Intraocular pressure (IOP) measurement
   Pupil dilation
   Binocular indirect ophthalmology and Fundus biomicroscopy
   Post-dilation IOP measurement
Counselling

the presenting complaint of the patient. Some optometrists perform direct ophthalmoscopy before the refraction.

Other test procedures should be inserted at appropriate times when the test result is not jeopardised by a preceding test and will not jeopardise tests that follow it in the eye examination.

Case history

The case history (case Hx) is the cornerstone of an optometric examination. Undoubtedly it can differentiate an experienced clinician from a novice. It is common for clinical supervisors to have to ask several additional questions of a patient after a student has completed the examination. Students should not worry about this as you will improve with experience! However, do not underestimate the value of history taking. There is much to learn about what questions should be asked and how much information can be gleaned from a proper history investigation.

- The case history allows a general observation of the patient (Px), e.g. Px's gait, head position, facial asymmetry, skin colour, physiological appearance in relation to chronological age, ability to speak and articulate, intellectual level, emotional state, assessment of overall state of health.
- Age, gender and race information allows you to think about the most likely problems knowing the prevalence of ocular disorders and their association with age, gender and race.
- Knowing the Px's chief complaint allows you to mentally list the most likely tentative diagnoses and ask appropriate supplementary questions to begin differential diagnosis during the case Hx. Some diagnoses (Dx) may rely heavily on case Hx, e.g. red eye, malingering, ocular hysteria.
- Case Hx provides information about the Px's happiness with his or her current spectacles/contact lenses. This information is heavily relied upon in the decision of whether to prescribe new lenses when the refractive change is low. Similarly, the degree of symptoms (Sxs), combined with your assessment of personality and the amount of detailed visual work performed, is very important in the decision of whether to prescribe a low-power refractive correction (Rx).
- The ocular history indicates whether the Px has had previous ocular treatment or surgery. An Hx of an ocular abnormality allows you to look for the manifestations of the disorder and any secondary effects (e.g. neovascular glaucoma with central retinal vein occlusion, etc.).
- The medical Hx may indicate that you should look particularly for ocular disorders which commonly manifest in certain systemic disease (most commonly diabetes) and whether it is safe to use certain Dx drugs (e.g. phenylephrine). The medication information may alert you to possible adverse effects of systemic medications (a common example being dry eye in an elderly hypertensive taking beta-blockers).
- Large increases in the likelihood of a Px with an affected first degree relative having certain systemic or ocular abnormalities means that you must look very carefully for appropriate signs/Sxs in Pxs with certain family ocular and medical histories (e.g. diabetes, hypertension, glaucoma, etc.).

- The Px's occupation and hobbies are very useful information when prescribing and counselling. For example, does the reading addition need to provide clear vision for computer work, reading, sewing or all three? Do they use protective eyewear when playing sports? It can also be important to know whether or not the Px drives with spectacles.
- Using the problem-oriented examination means that the case Hx decides to some degree which tests/procedures you are going to perform.

Finally, remember that your Px is a person and not a 'case'. Try to avoid being aloof and believe that your technical expertise can provide all the answers. It cannot. Patients want you to listen to them and to solve their problem(s), not to have you provide a diagnosis. It is essential to be a good listener, and to be interested in what the patients have to say. Give them the opportunity to describe all their visual and ocular problems.

Procedure

1. There should be full room illumination. Room lights should be on before the patient enters the examination room.
2. Observe the Px's appearance. Observe stature, walking ability and overall physical appearance. For example, a thin, 'twitchy' patient may have an overactive thyroid, an overweight, ruddy-faced and slightly sweaty older patient may be hypertensive, and type II diabetics are often slightly obese. Pay particular attention to any head tilt or obvious abnormalities of the face, eyelids and eyes that will require further investigation (such as facial asymmetry, acne, lid lesions, epiphora, entropion, ectropion, a red eye or strabismus).
3. The patient and clinician should be seated about 1 m apart at eye level. The examiner should face the patient and assume intermittent eye contact. The examiner should have the examination record card and record the history as the questions are being asked.
4. Chief complaint (CC). Determine the chief complaint by asking a very general open-ended question such as: 'Why have you come to see me today, Mr Jones?'; 'Is there any particular reason for your visit Ms Smith?'; or 'Do you have any problems with your vision or your eyes?'. A complete description of any complaint must be recorded (the order is given to provide a reasonable acronym LOFT SEA rather than a logical sequence):

    (a) Location/laterality: where is the problem located? Is it in both eyes or just one?
    (b) Onset: when did the problem begin?
    (c) Frequency/occurrence: how often does it occur? How long do the symptoms last?
    (d) Type/severity: obtain a relevant description, e.g. throbbing, sharp or dull headache, constant or intermittent blur, partial or total vision loss

(e) Self treatment and its effectivity: what makes the problem go away, if anything, and how well does it work?

(f) Effect on the patient: what has he or she done about it? Has the GP been seen? Is reduced vision affecting the patient's desired lifestyle?, etc.

(g) Associated factors: are there any other symptoms or other factors associated with the problem?

5. Symptom check. In patients stating they have no complaints to the general question asked above and just wish a check-up, ask about:

- Distance vision
- Near vision
- Double vision
- Eyestrain
- Headaches
- Pain and burning/discomfort

In a Px who has a CC, only ask about those aspects which were not described in the patient's CC. A complete description of any problem must be recorded (use the acronym LOFT SEA as above).

6. Ocular Hx:

(a) Ask about the Pxs' spectacles:

(i) When do they wear spectacles?
(ii) Age of the habitual spectacles?
(iii) Satisfaction with function/fashion of current spectacles?
(iv) Who prescribed the lenses?
(v) Age when glasses first worn?

(b) Ask about the Px's contact lenses: the type of lens worn, e.g. soft, hard, toric, bifocal, etc.; type of material, if known, e.g. PMMA, RGP, etc.; number of years lenses have been worn; age of current lenses; who prescribed the lenses and where the lenses were obtained; average wearing time, maximum wearing time, and time worn that day; solutions and cleaning regime; vision and symptoms with lenses (e.g. stinging, burning, irritation, discharge).

(c) Ask whether the patient has had any previous eye injuries, infections, surgery or treatment.

7. General health information. A general question of "How is your general health?" can be misleading because some patients think that systemic diseases are not relevant when they are borderline or are controlled by medication. It is better to follow up the initial question and give some examples of what is being specifically sought after, such as "Any high blood pressure or diabetes?". Another alternative is to ask whether the patient is under any medical care for anything (this can be a useful question to ask a female who may be pregnant). In addition, it is important to ask patients if they are taking any medication even if they indicate that their general health is fine.

Patients may believe their general health is fine because it is controlled by medication. Patients may also be taking medications but are unsure why, because the medical diagnosis was not properly explained or was poorly understood. Female patients may not consider birth control pills to be medication, yet as the drugs in these pills can have adverse ocular effects, it can be useful to ask about them specifically. Allergies and hypersensitivities to drugs or any other ingredients of medications or foodstuffs should also be ascertained at this point.

8. Family history. An open-ended question such as "Has anybody in your family had any eye problem or disease?" should be asked. This can be clarified by providing examples such as glaucoma or a lazy eye. Similarly, ask as 'Has anybody in your family had any medical problem such as diabetes or high blood pressure?'.

9. Health care. Determine when was the last eye examination (LEE) and by whom it was done, and when was the last medical examination (LME) and by whom it was done.

10. Vocation, sports, hobbies and driving. Record the visual demands, including lighting, visual posture, working distance and safety hazards/protection for the patient's vocation, as well as sports and hobbies. Record whether the patient drives and whether he or she wears contact lenses or spectacles when driving.

11. Remember that a case Hx continues throughout the examination. Certain signs or test results during the examination may suggest the need for further questioning.

Recording

Both positive and negative patient responses must be recorded. Remember that, from a legal viewpoint, if the response was not recorded the question was not asked. Avoid personal abbreviations. See Table 1.3.

Example

12-year-old Px Caucasian.
"Can't see blackboard" c̄ Rx last 6/12, gradual onset. TV = OK s̄Rx, sits close. NV = OK. No h/a. No other Sxs. Wears Rx for School only (B/ board, not outside). 1st wore age 10, this Rx 2 years old. Fashion = OK. GH = OK, no meds. No allergies.
No FOH, FMH: mum has IDDM.
LEE: 2 years, Mr. Smith's, Bradford.
LME: 6/12, Dr Jones, Bradford.

Interpretation: differential diagnosis

Once all verbal information is accurately collected the examiner should have a list of tentative diagnoses in mind for each of the identified

Table 1.3 Common abbreviations used in recording the case history

Px (or Pt)	Patient	Rx	Prescription
DS	Sphere	DC	Cylinder
CC	Chief complaint	DV	Distance vision
NV	Near vision	h/a	Headache
R	Right	L	Left
RE (or OD)	Right eye	LE (or OS)	Left eye
B (or binoc)	Binocular	BE	Both eyes
c̄	With	s̄	Without
1/52, 3/52	1 week, 3 weeks	3/12, 6/12	3 months, 6 months
↑	Increase	↓	Decrease
OK	Okay	Sx	Symptoms
FOH	Family ocular history	FMH	Family medical history
GH	General health	meds.	Medication
LEE	Last eye examination	LME	Last medical examination
Occ.	Ointment	Gutt.	Drops
B.D.	Twice a day	T.D.S.	Three times a day

problems. The remainder of the examination is based on testing to differentiate which of the tentative diagnoses is correct, as well as gathering essential database information.

Most common errors

1. Not fully investigating the patient's chief complaint.
2. Not recording all information obtained from the patient.
3. Failing to identify a drug name and dosage or identify possible side effects.
4. Not following through the case history in an organised manner.
5. Forgetting that case history taking can continue throughout the examination.
6. Taking the confidential case history in public (e.g. waiting room).
7. Assuming the same information is still current from the previous case history.
8. Recording personal abbreviations that will not be universally understood.
9. Repeating questions.
10. Leaving a record card on view to the public, such as on the reception desk.

Further reading

Amos, J.F. (1991). Patient history. In *Clinical Procedures in Optometry* (J.B. Eskridge, J.F. Amos and J.D. Bartlett, eds) J.B. Lippincott, Philadelphia, Pennsylvania

Elliott, D.B. (1997). The problem-oriented examination's case history. In *The Ocular Examination: Measurements and Findings* (K. Zadnik, ed.) W.B. Saunders, London, UK

2
Preliminary tests

Distance visual acuity

Background

Visual acuity (VA) is a measure of the patient's ability to resolve fine detail. It is the most commonly used measurement of visual function made by clinicians. VA is used to assess the adequacy of spectacle corrections and as a key indicator of ocular health. Visual acuity is also the criterion for a person's fitness to drive and ability to gain entrance into some professions. The need to measure VA accurately is obvious.

There are three principal measures of VA: unaided VA (vision), habitual VA (with the patient's own spectacles) and optimal VA (with the best refractive correction, i.e. after subjective refraction). VA with the retinoscope result is also often recorded. Either vision and/or habitual VA should be measured immediately after the case Hx for legal reasons, to document the VA level prior to your examination. Habitual and optimal distance VA are routine measurements. Measuring distance vision is optional, and should be measured with patients who do not wear spectacles, patients who have lost/broken their spectacles so that you cannot measure habitual VA (Professional Qualifying Examination [PQE] students note that in the routine examination section all 'patients' have lost their glasses), patients who do not wear spectacles for all or certain distance viewing tasks (this information must therefore be obtained in the case history), or if it is required for a report. Vision should also be measured if you suspect that the spectacle wearer may not really need to wear their spectacles all the time for distance and yet does so (does the young low hyperope need to wear the Rx at distance?). Measuring visual acuity after retinoscopy is particularly important in latent hyperopes where you need to know (and record) the level of distance vision blur with their manifest refractive correction.

Recommended test: Snellen visual acuity

Procedure

1. Leave the room lights on and illuminate the Snellen chart. The illuminance of the chart should be between 80 and 320 cd/m^2.

Rationale

The Snellen chart is widely available and used. A Snellen chart with a 'bottom line' of 6/3 is preferred, so that a true visual acuity can be measured (see interpretation). When they are available, logMAR visual acuity charts using the design principles suggested by Bailey and Lovie (e.g. 5 letters per line, 0.1 logMAR progression) are the chart of choice as they provide much more reliable indications of VA, particularly in patients with reduced VA. Unfortunately, at present they are not as widely available as they ought to be. When examining special populations (e.g. children, amblyopes, low vision patients), other charts and procedures should be used.

2. Seat the patient comfortably with an unobstructed view of the test chart. You should sit in front and to one side of the patient in order to monitor facial expressions and reactions.

3. If you are going to measure both vision and habitual VA, measure vision first to avoid memorisation. To measure vision ask the patient to remove any spectacles. To measure habitual visual acuity, ask the Px to put on his or her distance vision spectacles. Optimal visual acuity is measured after the subjective refraction.

4. Measure the visual acuity of the 'poorer' eye first, if a poorer eye is known from previous records or from the case history (to avoid a patient memorising the letters with the good eye and giving a false visual acuity with the poorer eye). Otherwise, measure VA in the right eye first.

5. Explain what measurement you are about to take. This can be as simple as "Now we shall find out what you can see".

6. Instruct the patient: "Please cover up your left/right eye with the palm of your hand/this occluder". If using the patient's hand, make sure that the palm is being used as otherwise the patient may be able to peek through fingers.

7. Ask the Px: "Please read the smallest line that you can see on the chart".

8. Continually monitor the patient's facial expressions. Do not permit the patient to screw up his or her eyes or look around the occluder or through fingers. (NB you need to be totally familiar with the test chart.)

9. Once the patients have reached what they believe is the smallest letters they can see, they should be pushed to determine whether they can see any more. Use prompts such as "Can you see any letters on the next line?", or "Have a guess. It doesn't matter if you get any wrong". Some patients are more cautious than others and only indicate those letters which they can see easily and clearly. Unless you push patients to guess, you could obtain different VA results depending on how cautious your patient is.

10. If the patient cannot see the largest letter on the chart, ask them to move closer to the letter until it is just recognised (or bring a large 60 m letter towards the patient until it is recognised). The distance at which this occurs should be noted.

11. If the patient cannot see the letters even at the closest test distance, use the following test sequence. Stop at the level at which the patient can accurately respond.

    (a) Count fingers (CF) @ X cms: the Px can count fingers at a certain distance.

    (b) Hand movements (HM) @ Y cms: the Px can see a hand moving from a certain distance.

    (c) Light projection (L proj.): the Px can report which direction light is coming from when you hold a pen light about 50 cm away. Ask the patient to point to the light and note the areas of the field in which the patient has light perception.

(d) Light perception (LP): the Px can see the light but not where it is coming from. If he or she cannot see light, the vision is recorded as no light perception or NLP.

12. Record vision/VA as the smallest line in which the majority of letters are read. Append errors with a plus (+) or minus (−) notation (see Recording below).
13. Repeat measurements for the other eye and binocularly.

Recording

Vision or visual acuity is recorded as the smallest line in which the majority of the letters are seen, irrespective of subjective blur. Errors are recorded by appending a minus one, two or three to the Snellen fraction, e.g. $6/9^{-2}$, $6/5^{-1}$, $6/5^{-3}$.

If additional letters are seen on the following line the Snellen fraction can be appended by a plus (usually up to no more than 3), e.g. $6/12^{+1}$, $6/6^{+3}$.

The Snellen fraction is defined as:

Test distance (m)/distance (m) at which the letters subtend 5 min of arc.

If the patient could not see the 6/60 letter at 6 m, but could at 2 m, record 2/60.

Interpretation

An optimal VA of 6/6 is often *considered* to be normal. It is, but only for the average patient over 50 years of age. Most young patients (and many older ones) have a visual acuity better than 6/6, and many young patients have VAs of 6/4 and even 6/3. It is important to use Snellen charts which measure down to 6/3, otherwise a slight drop in VA (from 6/3 or 6/4 to 6/6), which could indicate early ocular pathology or uncorrected refractive error, could be missed. If you have a chart with a bottom line of 6/5 or 6/6, be aware that a young patient could have 6/3 VA in one or both eyes, and complain of reduced VA even though they can see your 'bottom line'.

Note any deviation from normal age-matched results. Note any change from previous results. Note any interocular asymmetry, or binocular result that is *worse* than the monocular response.

For low myopic refractive errors, a degradation of one line of vision corresponds to approximately −0.25 D of refractive error, e.g. a −1.00 D myope with an optimal VA of 6/4 should have vision of 6/9 or 6/12. Near horizontal and vertical astigmatic errors have a similar effect to the equivalent best mean sphere, i.e. a −1.00 cyl would have a similar effect to a −0.50 DS, i.e. a 2-line drop in VA. Cylinders at oblique axes tend to give a slightly greater degradation in vision.

Because changes in astigmatism with age are negligible over the typical 1–4 year period between eye examinations, habitual VA reductions in spectacle wearing myopes and myopic astigmats indicate the increase in spherical power required, e.g. a myope of $-1.00/-1.00 \times 175$ with an habitual VA of 6/12 is likely to need a refractive correction of approximately $-2.00/-1.00 \times 175$. This rule can be used to check the accuracy of a subjective refraction result in myopes (and older hyperopes with no accommodation). By comparing habitual and optimal VA and using the rule one line of VA is equivalent to -0.25 DS, an estimate of the change in spherical Rx from the spectacles is gained. If this estimate is widely different from the actual subjective result, an error may be suspected and the subjective (and/or focimeter result) rechecked. If significant differences are found between the astigmatism in the spectacles and subjective refraction, an error in the focimetry and/or subjective refraction or a pathological change in astigmatism (due to e.g. keratoconus, chalazion, cataract) may be suspected.

Most common errors

1. Allowing the patients to decide their acuity (i.e. not 'pushing' them to guess).
2. Permitting the patients to screw their eyes up.
3. Permitting the patients to look around the occluder or through their fingers.
4. Using a low illumination (dirty chart and old bulb).
5. Using a wrong working distance – not 6 m.
6. Not recording the result immediately and guessing the result at the end of the examination.

Further reading

Bailey, I.L. (1997). Visual acuity. In *Clinical Refraction* (W.J. Benjamin and I. Borish, eds) W.B. Saunders, London, UK
Bullimore, M.A. (1997). Visual acuity. In *The Ocular Examination: Measurements and Findings* (K. Zadnik, ed.) W.B. Saunders, London, UK

Near visual acuity

Background

If we adhere to strict definitions, near visual acuity (VA) is rarely measured in clinical practice. Most of the tests of near VA do not use letter chart formats similar to those used for distance VA. Instead tests use sentences or paragraphs of words rather than isolated letters. They should perhaps be called reading tests. Reading tests measure a more complex function than VA and some patients (e.g. patients with age-related maculopathy [ARM] and amblyopia) are likely to have a reading acuity that is significantly worse than a near isolated-letter VA. In addition, reading charts are severely truncated as the smallest print usually shown, N5, only relates to a distance VA of about 6/9 when used at 40 cm.

Therefore they do not measure an acuity threshold and are really just a measure of the adequacy of a patient's reading ability: can they see well enough to be able to read print in the real world?

There are three principal measures of reading acuity or 'near VA': unaided near VA (near vision); habitual near VA (with the patient's own spectacles); and optimal near VA (with the best refractive correction). Habitual and optimal near VA are routine measurements in presbyopes and on all patients who complain of near vision problems. Measuring near vision is optional, and should be measured with presbyopic patients who do not wear spectacles for all or certain near viewing tasks (this information must therefore be obtained in the case history), or if it is required for a report. Reading acuity cannot always be assumed from distance visual acuity. For example, uncorrected presbyopes can have 6/5 in the distance and read only N12 or less on the near chart. A near VA should always be accompanied by a reading distance, as N10 at 40 cm is a totally different near VA to N10 at 10 cm.

Recommended test: N-notation near card using sentences

Procedure

1. Seat the patient comfortably with an unobstructed view of the near vision card. Sit in front and to one side of the patient in order to monitor facial expressions and reactions.
2. Keep the room lights on. *Do not* routinely use additional anglepoise lighting. Although this is commonly advocated, it is not always the situation used by the patient. In addition, given that N5 at 40 cm is far from a threshold measurement (see Interpretation below), increasing the illumination makes the test even easier. It may be better to restrict the use of anglepoise lighting to patients who indicate that they use such lighting when performing near tasks, and any patients who cannot easily read N5 in their optimal near refractive correction without additional lighting. These latter patients must be encouraged to obtain an anglepoise light for near tasks.
3. Instruct the patient to place the near vision card at his or her normal near working distance. Measure and record this distance (the Mallett unit has a very useful measuring device for this purpose).
4. Measure the near VA of the 'poorer' eye first, if a poorer eye is known from previous records or from the case history. Otherwise, measure the right eye first. Use an occluder or the patient's palm of the hand to cover the other eye. If using the patient's hand, make sure that the palm is being used, as otherwise the patient may be able to peek through his or her fingers.
5. Explain to the patient what measurement you are about to take. This may be a simple "Now we shall find out what you can see close up".
6. Instruct the patient to read the smallest paragraph he or she is able to read.

Rationale

N-print uses the New Times Roman font and is the standard test in the UK and widely available. It has a linear scale in that N10 is twice the size of N5, and can therefore be used effectively in low vision examinations to estimate required magnification. Most N-scale charts consist of sentences or passages of words which are more representative of real reading tasks. Charts which use a series of unrelated words are less representative of such tasks, but do avoid the patients using context to help them guess at some words.

M-unit charts are commonly used in North America and are as useful as N-scale charts. Jaeger notation should be avoided as there is no standardisation of what J1 or J5, etc. means. Different charts can give totally different sizes of print with the same J-value!

7. Unless the patient can see N5, push to determine whether he or she can see any more. Prompts such as "Try and make out some of the words on the smaller paragraph" may be useful. Some patients are more cautious than others and only indicate those letters which they can see easily and clearly. Unless you push patients to guess, you could obtain different near VA results depending on the cautiousness of your patient.
8. Repeat measurements for the left eye and binocularly.

Recording

Note the working distance and then record the paragraph size in N-notation for RE, LE and BE. For approximate equivalents to other notations see Table 2.1. Some clinicians do not note the working distance unless it is different from the 'norm'. Unfortunately even patients with good vision can present a wide range of normal working distances (25 cm to 50 cm) and, as stated earlier, a reading acuity is meaningless without a working distance.

Interpretation

Note any deviation from the normal level and any interocular differences. Near visual acuity is commonly measured only to N5, so that N5 at 40 cm is commonly accepted as being a normal level of near vision. This is incorrect. N5 at 40 cm is equivalent to about 6/9 distance VA. A patient could have 6/9 or even 6/12 distance VA and still have N5 at near. Realise that N5 is not a threshold measure and is used to give an indication of the adequacy of vision for reading most print sizes that patients will encounter. When determining a reading add, do not assume you have the correct add just because they can see N5.

Table 2.1   Near visual acuity equivalents

N-Notation 40 cm	Common usage	M-notation 40 cm	Point notation 40 cm	J notation 40 cm
3	Medicine bottle labels	0.4	3	—
4	Stock market print	0.5	4	1
5	Footnotes	0.6	5	2
6	Telephone directories	0.8	6	3
8	Small column newsprint	1.0	8	5
10	Typewritten	1.2	9	7
13	Books age 9–12 years	1.6	12	10
16	Computer display (80 column)	2.0	14	—
20	Books age 7–8 years	2.5	18	12
24	Large print books	3.0	—	14
32	Subheadlines	4.0	24	15
65	Newspaper headlines	8.0	—	16

Near visual acuity can be expected to be the same as distance visual acuity in most cases, provided that the eye is accommodating normally or that the reading addition is correct. There are some notable exceptions: pupil constriction with convergence causes the pupil area to become more completely filled in patients with posterior subcapsular cataract and near VA can be significantly less than distance VA. Patients with some eye disorders, such as amblyopia, ARM and macular oedema can have significantly worse reading VA than distance VA (and isolated-letter near VA).

Most common errors

1. Not recording the test distance.
2. Not watching the patients to see if they are screwing their eyes up or looking at the chart with both eyes.
3. Using a dirty near vision chart.
4. Using a reading test on an illiterate patient.

Further reading

Bailey, I.L. (1997). Visual acuity. In *Clinical Refraction* (W.J. Benjamin and I. Borish, eds) W.B. Saunders, London, UK

Bullimore, M.A. (1997). Visual acuity. In *The Ocular Examination: Measurements and Findings* (K. Zadnik, ed.) W.B. Saunders, London, UK

Classification of ocular deviations

The sensory and motor fusion mechanisms ensure the correct alignment of the eyes under binocular viewing conditions. If sensory fusion is prevented (for example; by occlusion on one eye), motor fusion will be frustrated and a deviation of the visual axes will occur in most patients. If the deviation is eliminated by the motor fusion reflex when the obstacle to sensory fusion is removed, the deviation is latent, and is called *heterophoria*.

If the fusion reflex fails to develop or is unable to function normally, the deviation of the eyes will be manifest and is called a *heterotropia* (squint, strabismus).

- A heterophoria is a latent deviation of the eyes.
- A heterotropia is a manifest deviation of the eyes.

Heterophoria

Classification of heterophoria with respect to direction of deviation

If the visual axes remain correctly aligned when sensory fusion is prevented the condition is known as ORTHOPHORIA.

If the visual axes deviate from alignment when sensory fusion is prevented the following conditions result:

- Converegence of the visual axes is called ESOPHORIA
- Divergence of the visual axes is called EXOPHORIA
- One visual axis higher than the other is called HYPERPHORIA
- One visual axis lower than the other is called HYPOPHORIA

Classification of vertical heterophorias is rather artificial. If the right axis is higher than the left this may be classified as either a right hyperphoria or a left hypophoria as it is difficult to determine which eye is correctly aligned. In practice, it is usual to classify vertical heterophorias as hyperphoria with deviations being recorded as either right hyperphoria or left hyperphoria to indicate the higher visual axis.

A relative rotation of the vertical poles of the cornea is called a cyclophoria. Deviation of the upper poles of the cornea result in the following:

- Outward rotation is known as EXCYCLOPHORIA
- Inward rotation is known as an INCYCLOPHORIA

Orthophoria is considered the ideal state rather than the normal state as most patients have a slight amount of heterophoria. At distance between 2^Δ of esophoria to 4^Δ of exophoria is considered normal. At near between 3 to 6^Δ of exophoria would be considered normal (physiological exophoria). The tolerance on vertical heterophoria is less than horizontal with only 0.5^Δ considered as normal.

Classification of heterophoria with respect to its effect on the vergence system

Convergence insufficiency: exophoria much larger at near than at distance.
Convergence excess: esophoria larger at near than at distance.
Divergence insufficiency: esophoria larger at distance than at near.
Divergence excess: exophoria larger at distance than at near.

Heterotropia (squint or strabismus)

Heterotropia (squint or strabismus): Classification with respect to direction of deviation

Heterotropia is classified with respect to the direction of deviation. If the visual axes deviate from alignment the following conditions result:

- Convergence of the visual axes is called ESOTROPIA
- Divergence of the visual axes is called EXOTROPIA
- If one visual axis points upwards it is called HYPERTROPIA
- If one visual axis points downwards it is called HYPOTROPIA

It is meaningful to classify vertical heterotropias as hyper or hypo as one eye will fixate whilst the other deviates either upwards or downwards. The heterotropia is signified by the direction of the non-fixating eye (for example: right hypotropia).

A rotation of the vertical poles of the cornea is called a cyclotropia. Deviation of the upper poles of the cornea result in the following:

- Outward rotation is known as an EXCYCLOTROPIA
- Inward rotation is known as an INCYCLOTROPIA

Concomitant and incomitant (paralytic) heterotropia

Incomitant heterotropia. A heterotropia in which the angle of deviation varies with direction of gaze. The angle of deviation is largest when the eyes are turned in the direction of maximum action of the affected muscle. The size of the deviation also varies with respect to the eye which is used to fixate. The primary angle of deviation is observed when the non-affected eye fixates. The secondary angle of deviation is observed when the affected eye fixates. The secondary angle is usually larger than the primary angle in recently aquired incomitancy.

The term 'paralysis' is used if the action of one or a group of extra-ocular muscles is completely abolished. If the action of a muscle is impaired but not abolished the term 'paresis' is used.

Concomitant heterotropia. A heterotropia in which the angle of deviation is constant in all directions of gaze. There are considerable variations in the type of concomitant heterotropia observed in clinical practice.

The deviation may be constant or intermittant as patients with limited fusional ability may be able to control the heterotropia some of the time. Under conditions of visual stress the fusional system breaks down allowing the deviation to become manifest. Cyclic heterotropia is a form of intermittant strabismus in which the deviation becomes manifest at regular intervals.

Unilateral heterotropia is one in which the patient constantly fixates with the same eye. Alternating heterotropia refers to patients who can use either eye to fixate. These patients usually have approximately equal VA in each eye.

Patients may present with a heterophoria at one fixation distance and a heterotropia at a different fixation distance. For example a patient with a high AC/A ratio may have a small esophoria at distance and an esotropia at near resulting in convergence excess. This is a concomitant condition and indicates an anomaly of the vergence system.

Classification of heterotropia in relation to the presence or absence of an accommodative component is of importance. Non-accommodative deviations are independent of the amount of accommodation being exerted. Accommodative or Donders squints increase in size when accommodative effort is exerted. There is usually a refractive component to this condition which can be corrected if the full refractive correction is prescribed.

25

Congenital strabismus is used to describe deviations which are present at birth or develop during the first few months of life. Acquired strabismus is applied to deviations which arise during childhood or later in life.

Further reading

Ciuffreda, K.J., Levi, D.M. and Selenow, A. (1991). *Amblyopia: Basic and Clinical Aspects*. Butterworth–Heinemann, Oxford, UK

Stidwell, D. (1990). *Orthoptic Assessment and Management*. Blackwell Scientific Publications, Oxford, UK

van Noorden, G.K. (1980). *Binocular Vision and Ocular Motility: Theory and Management of Strabismus*. C.V. Mosby, St. Louis, Missouri

Binocular status in the primary position

Background

An assessment of binocular status in the primary position is required at both distance and near to determine whether a heterotropia or heterophoria is present. If present, the direction, size, constancy and control of the deviation should be determined. It is usually important to determine the effect of any refractive error on the deviation, so the assessment of binocular status is often required in the unaided state and/or the patient's own spectacles and with the optimal refractive error.

Recommended test: Cover test

Procedure

1. Keep the room lights on and, if necessary, use localised lighting so that the patient's eyes can be easily seen with no shadows.
2. Seat the patient comfortably with his or her head erect and eyes in the primary position of gaze for the distance cover test. For the near cover test, the eyes should be in a slight downward gaze.
3. Explain the procedure to the patient: "I am now going to find out how well your eye muscles work together".
4. Isolate a single letter of a size equal to or slightly larger than the patient's visual acuity of the poorer eye. It is important to select a target which will act as an accommodative stimulus if possible. If the monocular visual acuity in the poorer eye is less than 6/18, use a spot light for fixation. Using a letter larger than 6/18 for fixation usually results in unsteady fixation as the patient scans the letter. Although the spotlight is not an accommodative stimulus, it is a reasonable compromise for patients with poor vision or VA. At near, use a single isolated letter of a size equal to or slightly larger than the near visual acuity of the poorer eye.

5. Instruct the patient: "I would like you to look at the letter * at the other end of the room (or the letter * on this stick). Please keep your eyes on the letter as I place this cover in front of your eye. If the letter appears to move please follow it with your eyes".

6. First perform the cover/uncover test to look for a heterotropia (Figure 2.1): place the cover before one eye and then remove it, allowing both eyes to fixate the target, if this is possible. The cover/uncover test gives a measure of the habitual angle of deviation.

   (a) Observe the response of the eye which has not been covered. If this eye moves when the other is covered, then a *heterotropia* is present in the moving eye. The movement observed is one to take up fixation. If the eye moves out to take up fixation, an ESOtropia is present. If the eye moves in to take up fixation, an EXOtropia is present.

   (b) Repeat the cover/uncover test by placing the cover over the other eye and look for a squint.

   (c) Repeat the test several times to ensure the correct diagnosis.

7. If a squint is not present, perform the cover/uncover test to look for a hetrophoria (Figure 2.2):

   (a) Observe the response of the occluded eye behind the occluder when it is first covered. If a heterophoria is present then the covered eye will drift outwards in EXOphoria, and inwards in ESOphoria.

   (b) If a heterophoria is present, observe the response of the occluded eye when the cover is removed. If a heterophoria is present, the previously covered eye will make a fusional recovery movement (outwards in ESOphoria and inwards in EXOphoria).

8. Perform the alternate cover test. The alternate cover test does *not* help distinguish between a heterophoria and heterotropia, but gives a measure of the total angle of deviation. It is useful when trying to place stress on the oculomotor system and can break a heterophoria down into a heterotropia.

   (a) Place the occluder before one eye and then transfer it from one eye to the other, so that at no time are both eyes allowed to fixate the target together.

   (b) If there is a deviation of the eyes, it will be seen as a re-fixation (saccadic) eye movement when the cover is transferred from one eye to the other.

   (c) Observe the latency and the speed of the fusional recovery movement on the final uncovering, since this may give clues as to the strength of the fusion reflex.

9. Estimate or measure the magnitude of the deviation. Estimates can be made with experience. Deviations can be measured by placing prisms of increasing power in front of one eye until no movement is observed

Rationale

The cover test is the only method by which an ocular deviation can be distinguished as either a heterotropia (also called a squint or strabismus) or a heterophoria. This test uses the simplest method of dissociating the eyes and removing the fusion reflex: covering one eye whilst the other fixates a target. The test has the advantage of being an objective test (i.e. one that does not require a response from the patient), although the subjective response of the patient while performing the test can provide valuable additional information. The cover test provides considerable information about the direction, size, stability and control of a deviation. It is quick and simple to perform but requires considerable practice before accurate observations can be made. A distance and near cover test should be performed on every patient. The test should be performed with the patient's habitual refractive correction in place and in some cases repeated without the refractive correction to allow the accommodative components of the condition to be assessed.

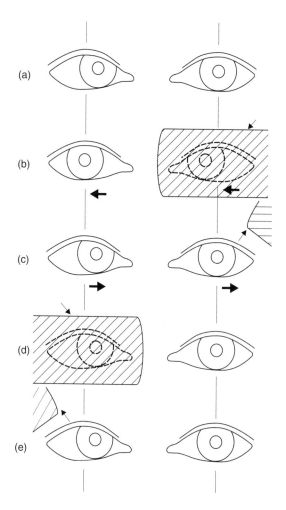

Figure 2.1 Cover test in a patient with a right esotropia. (a) The right eye deviates inwards slightly, but this may not be obvious depending on its size and your experience. (b) Cover the left eye and the right eye is seen to move out to take up fixation. Behind the cover the left eye moves to the right, obeying Hering's law. (c) Uncover the left eye and the left eye now moves out to take up fixation, as it is the dominant eye. The right eye moves to the left, obeying Hering's law. (d) Cover up the right eye and no movement occurs. (e) Uncover the right eye and no movement occurs. (Reprinted with permission from Pickwell, D. (1989) *Binocular Vision Anomalies*. Butterworth–Heinemann, Oxford, UK.)

with the cover test. Base-in prism is used to measure exophoria, and base-out to measure esophoria. A prism bar is most conveniently used for this purpose.

Recording

1. NMD (no movement detected) or 'ortho'.
2. If strabismus is detected, then record which eye is deviated (right, left, alternating), the constancy (intermittent, constant), the direction

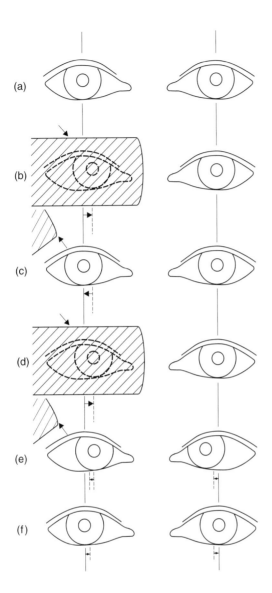

Figure 2.2 Cover test in a patient with esophoria: (a) to (c) show the simple pattern of eye movements which are usually seen, and (d) to (f) show the more rare versional pattern of movements which can occur when one eye is very dominant. (a) Both eyes look straight ahead. (b) Cover the right eye and the left eye does not move, indicating that there is no squint in the left eye. Behind the cover the right eye moves inwards. (c) Uncover the right eye and the left eye moves out to resume fixation with the other eye. Notice that during the movements of the right eye, the left eye has not moved, and disobeys Hering's law to maintain fixation. (d) Cover the right eye and the left eye does not move, indicating that there is no squint in the left eye. Behind the cover the right eye moves inwards. (e) Uncover the right eye and both eyes move right by the same amount, obeying Hering's law. (f) Both eyes diverge to the straight position. (Reprinted with permission from Pickwell, D. (1989). *Binocular Vision Anomalies*. Butterworth–Heinemann, Oxford.)

(exo, eso, right hyper, right hypo, left hyper, left hypo, excyclo, incyclo) and the suffix tropia (abbreviate to T, e.g. SOT, XOT). Also record an estimation of the size of the deviation, preceding your result with the symbol $\sim$ (e.g. $\sim 10^\Delta$ (XOT).

3. If the deviation is not constant, note the percentage of time that the eye deviates.
4. If heterophoria is detected, then record the direction (SOP, XOP, R/L) and magnitude of the deviation, and the nature of the recovery movement to binocular fixation.

Interpretation

Once the cover test has diagnosed a heterotropia or heterophoria, several subsequent procedures are required to provide further diagnostic information and information which may be of value when treating the condition (*see* Treatment of binocular vision anomalies).

Heterotropia

1. If a heterotropia is present it is essential to determine if the condition is incomitant or concomitant using a motility test. New incomitant deviations should be referred for further investigation (*see* Comitancy of an ocular deviation).
2. The presence of a heterotropia indicates that certain binocular vision tests such as Maddox rod and wing, fixation disparity and binocular balancing would provide no useful information. Indeed, using these tests on a patient with heterotropia indicates a lack of knowledge of the information provided by these tests.

Concomitant heterotropia

1. In children, a cycloplegic refraction should be conducted to ensure the full refractive error is measured. This is usually unnecessary in adults as their accommodative amplitude is smaller than children's and the full refractive error can be determined using retinoscopy.
2. Correction of fully accommodative heterotropia can be achieved by prescribing the full refractive error. Although this may initially reduce visual acuity it is important to prescribe the full correction to ensure binocularity. Treatment of any sensory anomaly should be considered. An important consideration for treatment of amblyopia is the patient's age.
3. In partially accommodative and non-accommodative heterotropia the size of the residual deviation should be measured. A heterotropia greater than about 15^Δ may be able to benefit from cosmetic surgery and this could be discussed with the patient or their guardian.
4. Eccentric fixation should be assessed to determine the relative extent of visual acuity loss due to eccentric fixation and amblyopia.

Heterophoria

1. Heterophorias are usually only investigated further if the patient has appropriate symptoms; if the heterophoria is large and/or has a poor

recovery, and if any subsequently found change in refractive error could produce a decompensated heterophoria.

2. In children, a cycloplegic refraction should be conducted to ensure the full refractive error is measured. This is usually unnecessary in adults as their accommodative amplitude is smaller than children's and the full refractive error can be determined using retinoscopy.

3. Compare the deviation present at distance and near as this relationship further diagnoses the heterophoria and can be of value in identifying a course of action.

4. The following measurements are frequently of value: fusional reserves, fixation disparity, near point of convergence and the AC/A ratio when deciding on treatment (see Treatment of binocular vision anomalies).

5. It can be useful to measure the amount of additional spherical lens power which neutralises fixation disparity as well as associated phoria.

Most common errors

1. Diagnosing as a strabismus the immediate loss and recovery of fixation of an eye when the other eye is covered. Because of a heterophoria movement of the covered eye during the covering process, the fixing eye may move from its original accurate foveal position due to Hering's law of equal innervation, and then refixate due to the fixation reflex.

2. Diagnosing the eye movements observed where a versional flick recovery is present as a strabismus. A version/vergence movement will often be seen as fusion is regained in the case where a high phoria is present (Figure 2.2).

3. Covering and uncovering the eyes so rapidly that the patient does not have adequate time to change fixation if required.

4. Not watching for an alternating strabismus when switching from covering–uncovering left eye to covering–uncovering right eye.

5. Using large sweeping lateral movement of the occluder when covering/uncovering. This is distracting and encourages eye movements. Small vertical movement with the occluder are all that is required.

6. Missing a strabismus in deep amblyopia by not choosing an appropriate fixation target and not actively encouraging fixation of the non-fixing eye.

Acceptable alternative procedure: Hirschberg test

Procedure

1. Keep the room fully illuminated. Additional use of localised lighting is recommended so that the patient's eyes can be seen easily with no shadow.

Rationale

The Hirschberg test is quick and easy to perform, requiring little cooperation on the part of the patient. It may be

31

the only test of binocularity possible with uncooperative patients such as young children and people with development disabilities. However, it can only be performed at near, provides a poor stimulus to accommodation and is relatively inaccurate. In addition, large angle lambdas may result in the misdiagnosis of pseudo-strabismus.

2. Ask the patient to remove any spectacles. If it is felt that the correction will alter the result, the test should also be performed through the correction.
3. Hold a pen light directly in front of your eyes and 40 to 50 cm from the patient.
4. Ask the patient to look at the light with both eyes open. Young children will tend to look toward the bright light but may need a little encouragement.
5. Note the location of the corneal reflex in each eye individually. Usually the reflex is decentred inward with respect to the centre of the pupil. This is a small positive angle lambda.
6. Note the location of the corneal reflexes as the patient views binocularly. The eye that has the same angle lambda as in the monocular test is the fixing eye. The location of that reflex should be considered the reference position.
7. The corneal reflex of the fellow eye will have shifted in a direction opposite to that of the ocular deviation.
8. Estimate the magnitude of the deviation by estimating the displacement of the reflex in mm relative to the reference position: $1 \text{ mm} = 12^{\Delta}$. If the reflex is positioned on the pupil margin, the deviation is approximately 40^{Δ}.

Recording

Record which eye deviates, along with the direction of the deviation. Note that the observation was made using the Hirschberg technique. Equal nasal displacement of the corneal reflexes in each eye indicates a non-strabismic patient.

Interpretation

A reflex located nasally to the reference point suggests an exotropia, a reflex located temporally to the reference point suggests an esotropia. Superior displacement of the reflex suggests a hypotropia, and inferior displacement suggests a hypertropia.

Most common errors

1. Not viewing directly behind the pen light.
2. Placing too much emphasis on this gross test.

Further reading

Pickwell, L.D. (1989). *Binocular Vision Anomalies*, 2nd edn. Butterworths, London, UK
Stidwell, D. (1990). *Orthoptic Assessment and Management*. Blackwell Scientific Publications, Oxford, UK

Comitancy of an ocular deviation

Background

It is essential to be able to distinguish between concomitant and incomitant deviations. An incomitant deviation is one in which the size of the deviation varies with direction of gaze. A concomitant deviation is one in which the angle of squint is constant for all directions of gaze for a given fixation distance.

Some patients present with no deviation at distance but an exotropia at near. This is *not* an incomitancy but results from an anomaly of the vergence mechanism.

Incomitant deviations can be due to a pathological cause or trauma and must be referred for a medical opinion if they are of recent onset. It is not only important to correctly diagnose an incomitancy but additionally it is essential to detect whether the condition is of recent onset or long-standing. Clearly, an old incomitancy is not in need of referral as the condition will have been investigated and treated previously. An incomitancy of recent onset requires immediate referral as the underlying causes are possibly serious. Patients with recent onset incomitancy complain of a rapid onset of diplopia and possible head tilt, a recent blow to the head and present with past-pointing (see Table 2.2).

Recommended test: Motility test

Procedure

1. Keep the room lights on.
2. Seat the patient comfortably with his or her head in the primary position. Patients should wear their own spectacles unless the frame is too small or the patient wears bifocals or varifocals. Sit directly in front of the patient so that both eyes can be viewed simultaneously.
3. Explain the measurement to the patient: "I am now going to determine whether your eye muscles work together in different positions of gaze".
4. Direct a pen torch at the patient's eyes. Observe the position of the corneal reflex in each eye.
5. Instruct the patient: "Please watch my light and follow it with your eyes. Keep your head still. Tell me if the light appears double or if your eyes are uncomfortable or if you cannot keep looking at the light for any reason".
6. Hold the pen torch approximately 50 cm from the patient and move it in an arc with the subject's head as centre. Stay in the binocular field (the loss of the corneal reflex can help to indicate that you are outside the binocular field).
7. Move the pen torch into the nine diagnostic positions of gaze by moving the target in a cross or H formation (Figure 2.3). Many

Rationale

This is the simplest method (but also the least sensitive) of evaluating a deviation in the nine diagnostic positions of gaze; it is by direct observation of the eyes as the patient fixates a pen light. This test is available to all clinicians as it is cheap and easy to perform.

Table 2.2 Signs and symptoms which can differentiate between old and new ocular muscle palsy

Sign or symptom	Old	New
Diplopia	Rare	Almost always present
Onset	Generally known	Probably sudden
Amblyopia	Common	Rare
Trauma	Not usual	Common
Symptoms	Not usual	Common and extreme
Comitance	Spread of concomitance may obscure original palsy	Always incomitant
Abnormal head posture	If present well established and difficult to alter	Can be marked but easy to alter. Covering paretic eye eliminates problem
Past-pointing	Absent	Present
Health	Not usually related	Current health may be a significant issue

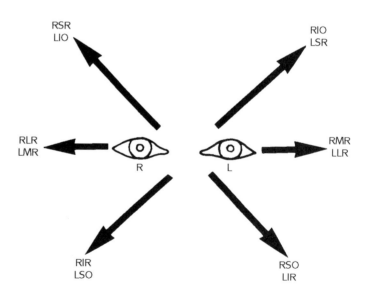

Figure 2.3 The six cardinal diagnostic positions of gaze, showing the extra-ocular muscles which maintain the eyes in these positions. (Reprinted with permission from Pickwell, D. (1989). *Binocular Vision Anomalies*. Butterworth–Heinemann, Oxford, UK.) Assessment of motility up and down the vertical midline is essential for the diagnosis of conditions such as A and V patterns. The three diagnositic positions on the midline supplement the six positions of fixation demonstrated in the diagram. LR = lateral rectus; MR = medial rectus; IR = inferior rectus; SR = superior rectus; SO = superior oblique; IO = inferior oblique.

clinicians have a preference in the manner in which the light is moved but either type of movement is acceptable.

8. Look for any misalignment of the eyes in all positions of gaze (the corneal reflexes may help you in this).
9. If diplopia is reported, determine if it is horizontal or vertical.
10. Locate the region of greatest diplopia as this indicates the direction in which the greatest underaction occurs.
11. Isolate the images to find out which eye sees which image. The image furthest away is that seen by the paretic eye (red/green goggles can help in locating the images). A cover test performed in this direction of gaze can help confirm the diagnosis.

Recording

Where the ocular movements appear full and no diplopia is reported in any position, a normal result has been obtained. In the case of a non-squinting patient, record this as 'Full co-ordinated movements', and for a patient with strabismus as 'No incomitancy'. Record any apparent under-actions or restrictions, clearly stating which eye and in which gaze direction.

Interpretation

If an eye cannot follow the object of regard as it is taken into all the positions of gaze, then there is an underaction or restriction of one or a combination of extra-ocular muscles (EOMs). To determine which EOM is affected consider the muscle actions (Figure 2.3).

To aid or confirm a diagnosis of the underaction/restriction and to measure the extent of the deviation, further tests are required, such as the Hess screen test (see Degree of incomitancy, Chapter 4).

Most common errors

1. Performing the test too quickly.
2. Not asking the patient to report doubling, or not fully investigating reported doubling.
3. Misinterpreting a large intermittent squint as an incomitancy.
4. Not maintaining full elevation across the upper motor field.
5. Allowing the subject to move his or her head.

Further reading

Pickwell, L.D. (1989). *Binocular Vision Anomalies*, 2nd edn. Butterworths, London, UK
Stidwell, D. (1990). *Orthoptic Assessment and Management*. Blackwell Scientific Publications, Oxford, UK

Convergence ability

Background

In a patient with normal binocular function, the ability of the eyes to converge when viewing a near visual task is paramount to the patient's visual comfort. They do so in response to muscle tonus, proximity of a near object and in synkinesis with accommodation. Many patients experience symptoms due to an inability to converge adequately, and it is important to measure this routinely.

Recommended tests: Near point of convergence (NPC) and Jump convergence

The jump convergence test is also useful clinically, as in normal vision we tend to change fixation distance in jumps. The patient is simply asked to change fixation between two discrete points and the near point determined. It is felt by some clinicians to provide an assessment of near vision which is more closely aligned to normal vision than the NPC. Jump convergence can be used as an additional assessment in patients who show a remote NPC to provide a more comprehensive assessment of convergence ability, and in patients with symptoms which could suggest convergence problems who show a normal NPC.

Near point of convergence (NPC)

Rationale.
The near point of convergence (NPC) is the point where the visual axes intersect under the maximum effort of convergence while binocular single vision is retained. It is the standard test for convergence ability and has the advantage over jump convergence in that it provides a quantitative assessment. It is also quick and easy to perform and requires little extra equipment.

Procedure

1. Seat the patient comfortably with his or her head erect and eyes in slightly downward gaze. Make sure the patient is wearing their near correction. Sit directly in front of the patient so that both eyes can be viewed simultaneously.
2. Keep the room lights on. Position the anglepoise light to illuminate the patient's eyes or the target (whichever is necessary) without shadows.
3. Explain the measurement to the patient: "This test determines how well your eyes can converge to a close object".
4. Position the target (the fine high contrast vertical line target on the RAF rule is useful) at a distance of 50 cm directly in front of the patient slightly below the midline.
5. Instruct the patient: "Please watch the line as I move it towards you and tell me if it goes double".
6. Make sure that the patient is looking at the target with *both* eyes.
7. Slowly and steadily move the target toward the bridge of the patient's nose. The speed should be such that it takes approximately 10 sec to move the target from 50 cm to the bridge of the patient's nose.
8. Watch the patient's eyes for loss of convergence (objective NPC). Measure the distance the target is from the eyes when one of the eyes loses fixation and/or the patient becomes aware of diplopia.

9. If the target becomes double (subjective NPC) before it is more than 12–15 cm from the bridge of the nose, encourage the patient to make an extra effort to make the target single again. Moving it away slightly will help this. If single binocular vision can be re-established advance the target again towards the patient.

10. For a remote NPC also move the target back and note the point of fusion.

11. If the history indicates that the patient requires prolonged and/or excessive convergence in a specific position of gaze then repeat the procedure in that specific position.

Recording. NPC should be recorded in centimetres from the bridge of the nose. For example, 12 cm right eye deviates with diplopia (shorten to 12 cm RE c̄ dip.). If the measurements are taken in any position other than the primary position then the gaze position must be recorded. If the eyes lose fixation by over-convergence (as in the case of an above-average AC/A ratio), then this should be noted. If there is obvious dissociation of the eyes with no reported diplopia by the patient, then possible suppression should be noted, and investigated further.

Interpretation. The pre-presbyope should be able to converge the eyes up to the bridge of their nose. If the eyes cannot converge up to at least 12–15 cm from the bridge of the nose, the patient has a reduced ability to converge the eyes. A normal response is approximately 8 cm. If one eye obviously dissociates but diplopia is not noted then suppression is present. The patient is less likely to suffer from symptoms due to the poor convergence.

Most common errors
1. Allowing the patient to confuse blurring for doubling.
2. Using an inappropriate target (e.g. a pen).
3. Testing the eyes in upward or primary gaze instead of slightly downward gaze.
4. Moving the target too rapidly and unsteadily.
5. Not pushing the patient enough to keep the target single.

Jump convergence

Procedure
1. Seat the patient comfortably with his or her head erect and eyes in slightly downward gaze. The patient should be corrected for distance. Sit directly in front of the patient so that both eyes can be viewed simultaneously, but so that distance fixation is not obscured.
2. Keep the room lights on. Position the anglepoise light to illuminate the patient's eyes or the target (whichever is necessary) without shadows.
3. Indicate clearly to the patient both a distant (Snellen letter) and near (fixation rule) target.

4. Position the near target about 40 cm in front of the patient, and ask him or her to alternate fixation from the distant target to the near target and back again.
5. Move the near target to 20 cm, and then 10 cm, repeating the procedure each time.
6. Continually watch that the eyes converge and diverge quickly and smoothly, and that binocular fixation is obtained each time.

Recording. Record the closest distance in centimetres to which a fast, smooth convergence is made, e.g. 'Jump convergence good to 10 cm'. Any other observations should be recorded, such as 'Jump convergence delayed and jerky, but achieves 10 cm', or 'Poor jump convergence to 30 cm'.

Interpretation. Good, fast, smooth jump convergence should be observed to 10–15 cm. If a normal result is not observed, the patient has a reduced ability to converge the eyes (convergence insufficiency). This must be assessed in the light of any symptoms.

Further reading

Pickwell, L.D. (1989). *Binocular Vision Anomalies*, 2nd edn. Butterworths, London, UK
Stidwell, D. (1990). *Orthoptic Assessment and Management.* Blackwell Scientific Publications, Oxford, UK

Testing for gross visual field defects

Background

A variety of simple visual field tests are available and include confrontation fields, kinetic boundary testing, colour comparison fields and oculokinetic perimetry (OKP). They are used to screen quickly and easily for relatively gross visual field defects. In any patient where there is an indication of a field defect (as suggested by symptoms, signs or risk factors) simple visual field testing is wholly inappropriate and a full quantification of threshold visual fields *must* be performed. The relative sensitivity of these simple visual field tests compared to automated visual field screening is not known. However, they have all been shown to be insensitive to field defects other than homonymous hemianopias when compared to the standard Goldmann or Humphrey visual field assessments. Their prime use is likely to be when an automated screener is not available and during domiciliary visits.

Recommended test: Confrontation fields using a 'bead on a stick'

Rationale

The 'routine' section of the PQE exams requires a confrontation or kinetic boundary examination to be performed. The preferred target for most examiners appears to be a circular white bead of about 4 mm diameter on the end of a black stick. A red bead of similar size at the other end of the stick can be useful if the back wall is white so that the white target is of very low contrast. Confrontation fields are preferred to kinetic boundary testing (where only the peripheral limits of the field are determined using the bead-on-a-stick, as in arc perimetry), as there are few ocular diseases which provide a peripheral field loss before a central field loss or a generalised constriction. Those that do (e.g. retinitis pigmentosa, retinal detachment and retinoschisis) should be detected by procedures other than confrontation fields (e.g. binocular indirect ophthalmoscopy). Field defects caused by chiasmal or post-chiasmal lesions are usually detectable within 30 degrees of fixation. Central field defects are always of greater clinical importance than any peripheral defects and plotting of the peripheral field alone is considered ineffective. In the few studies that have been performed, colour comparison fields have been shown to be more sensitive to field defects than confrontation fields using fingers as targets. However, at present these tests are rarely used in UK optometry.

Procedure

1. Explain to the patients that you are going to measure the area over which they can see rather than how well they can see detail.

2. Keep the room lights on. The absolute level is irrelevant as the technique involves a comparison of the patient's and examiner's visual fields.

3. Sit between 66 cm and 1 m away from, and directly facing, the patient. You should be at approximately the same height as the patient.

4. Ask the patient to remove any glasses and occlude his or her left eye using the palm of the hand (not fingers).

5. You should similarly occlude your right eye.

6. Ask the patient to fixate your open eye (left) with his or her open eye (right). Some patients may feel uncomfortable if asked to stare into your eye directly, and you can suggest they look at the middle of your lower lid.

7. Show the patient the bead-on-a-stick and explain that you are going to move it inwards from outside the field of view and you want the patient to indicate when he or she can first see the target. Explain that you will continue to move the target into the centre of the patient's vision and you want him or her to indicate if it disappears or fades at any point.

8. Hold the bead-on-a-stick in a plane equidistant between you and the patient and outside your field of view along one of the eight principal radial meridians. Slowly move the bead inwards until the patient reports it is just seen. Compare this point to the point when you first saw the target. Then slowly move the target towards fixation and ask the patient to indicate if it disappears or becomes less distinct.

9. Repeat this procedure for all eight radial meridians. At all times watch that the patient does not lose fixation of your eye to look towards the target. If this occurs, repeat the measurement.
10. Repeat for the other eye.

Recording

Record the type of confrontation target used and whether there were any significant differences between your own visual field and the patient's visual field. A normal result could be recorded as 'Fields full to confrontation, 4 mm W'.

Interpretation

Confrontation testing involves a comparison of your visual field with the patient's visual field. Providing there is no obvious abnormality in your field, the patient's field is considered within normal limits if it matches your own. Confrontation field testing provides the minimum visual field data for any given patient. It is useful in the detection of large absolute defects, e.g. quadrantanopsia and homonymous, heteronymous or altitudinal hemianopsia. It may even be possible to detect an advanced nasal step, although by that stage there would probably be many other indications of abnormality.

Most common errors

1. Not accurately comparing your visual field with the patient's visual field.
2. Using too cluttered a visual field (loud tie or blouse, wall picture, bookcase).
3. Using poor alignment for height.
4. Allowing the patient to lose fixation.
5. Believing that other visual field assessments are not necessary if confrontation does not show a defect.

Further reading

Elliott, D. B., North I. and Flanagan, J. G. (1997). Confrontation visual fields clinical optometry update. *Opthal. Physiol. Opt.* Suppl. (in press).

Colour vision testing

Background

Congenital colour deficiency is found in both eyes equally and does not change over time. It is virtually always a red–green deficiency and is far more common in males than females as it is an X-linked disorder: 8% (1 in 12) of the male and 0.5% of the female population are red–green deficient.

Due to the increased use of colour as a teaching aid in schools, it is important to perform colour vision screenings on children soon after the commencement of school. All hereditary colour defectives should be reassured about their condition: that they are not colour blind, that it is not a disease and that the condition will always remain but will not get worse. Young colour defectives and their parents should be counselled that their condition lessens their chances of joining certain occupations, such as the RAF, police force and the fire brigade. The more severe the colour deficiency, the more unlikely their chances of joining. In addition to these occupations, the presence of a colour deficiency results in greater difficulty in pursuing a career that stresses the ability to discriminate colour. Such careers include histology, chemistry, photography, the paint and textiles industries, interior decorating and electronics.

Acquired colour defects are normally monocular or unequal in the two eyes, found about equally in males and females, can progress (or regress) and most often involve a loss of blue sensitivity leading to blue–green and yellow–violet discrimination loss accompanied by decreased vision. Acquired defects may be due to the presence of an anomaly involving the internal components of the eye (lens, ocular media, retina), optic nerve or the visual pathways. These anomalies are secondary to ocular or systemic pathologies, drugs, or toxic substances. In patients with acquired colour deficiencies, their colour problems can get ignored because other aspects of vision, such as acuity or visual fields, are reduced and take precedent. Although these latter tests may be more routinely measured in patients with ocular abnormality and may be more important from a diagnostic perspective, colour vision is an important part of the assessment of a patient's real world vision. It can provide useful information in any patient with reduced vision due to ocular disease, and obviously in any patient who complains of colour vision problems. Particular examples of advice for patients with acquired colour vision defects include suggesting that diabetics with a colour deficiency monitor their blood sugar levels using blood-glucose tests rather than trying to differentiate the colours on urine-glucose tests. Similarly, elderly individuals should be warned of possible difficulty in differentiating certain coloured tablets.

Recommended tests: Ishihara pseudoisochromatic plates and The City University colour vision

Ishihara plates

Procedure

1. You must use the proper quantity and quality of illumination, as the colour temperature of the illuminant will affect the colours of the test. Colour vision testing is normally performed under a standard illuminant source C, in the form of the Macbeth Easel lamp. This simulates natural daylight conditions provided by direct sunlight and a clear sky. As the Macbeth Easel lamp is expensive, other alternative sources are often used. For example, you can use a Kodak Wratten #78AA filter

Rationale.

No single colour vision test is capable of screening, diagnosing, and grading the severity of acquired or congenital colour vision defects, and it is recommended that a test battery be used. When screening for congenital colour deficiency, a plate test such as the Ishihara should be used to help separate individuals with normal colour vision from those with a deficiency. The Ishihara remains the most efficient screening test for red–green colour deficiency. If a patient is determined to be colour deficient using the Ishihara plates, another test such as the City University colour vision test (TCU) or the Farnsworth D-15 (or desaturated D-15) should be used to grade the severity and classify the deficiency. Patients who fail the Ishihara and then pass the TCU or D-15 have a mild red–green defect, and are unlikely to have trouble with most occupations. When evaluating the extent and monitoring an acquired colour deficiency, the TCU or D-15 is recommended. The TCU test is probably the most useful test to use in the UK as it is widely available and has become the standard test for some police forces. *Special testing for occupational or vocational placement depends upon the individual vocational standards.*

(found in camera shops) placed in front of the patient's eye in conjunction with a 100 watt incandescent light source; or high colour rendering fluorescent lights (> 6400 K). Natural daylight is not recommended due to its variability in both the quality and quantity of light, although even this is preferable to tungsten lighting.

2. Explain to the patient that you are going to test colour vision.
3. If screening for a congenital defect, measure colour vision binocularly. If screening for an acquired defect, measure colour vision monocularly.
4. Ask the patient to use his or her near vision correction and hold the booklet at arm's length.
5. Ask the patient to read the numbers, starting at plate one. The patient should only be allowed about 3 sec to view each plate.

Recording. Ishihara: record the number of plates correctly determined out of the number of plates attempted, for example, 'Ishihara 16/20'. Do not include the demonstration plate in this recording.

Interpretation. Ishihara: plate 1 is a demonstration plate which should be read by all literate patients and can be used to indicate malingerers. Different designs of pseudoisochromatic plates follow, and include transformation (plates 2–9), vanishing (10–17) and hidden digit (18–21) plates. Normal trichromats can see numbers on all but the hidden digit plates. Patients with red–green colour deficiency do not see a number on the vanishing plates, see a different number to normals on the transformation plates and *can* see a number on the hidden digit plates. Classification plates, which attempt to differentiate protans and deutans, are found on plates 22–25. Two numbers are shown on each plate. The right hand number (blue–purple) is not seen or seen less well by deutans, and the left hand number (red–purple) is not seen or less well seen by protans. The rest of the plates contain isochromatic pathways and are used for patients who cannot read letters, such as young children. The patient's task is to trace the pathway.

Normals will make few, if any, mistakes. The pass/fail criteria are different for the various versions of the test, but this information is included in the test manual. Generally, any more than two incorrect plates constitutes a fail. Even though the Ishihara test is efficient at screening for red–green defects, it should not be used to classify the severity of a colour vision deficiency. Other limitations of this test include its inability to screen for tritan deficiencies and the fading of colours with time.

Most common errors
1. Assuming that using the Ishihara test alone is a sufficient assessment of a congenital colour deficiency.
2. Using an unsuitable light source.
3. Allowing the patient too long to look at the figures.

4. When screening a patient for a certain occupation or vocation, using a commonly used test such as the Ishihara rather than the test(s) specified in the appropriate vocational standards.
5. Attempting to assess an acquired colour deficiency using the Ishihara test.

The City University colour vision test

Procedure

1. Ensure you are using the correct lighting conditions (see above).
2. Explain to the patient that you are going to test colour vision.
3. If you are assessing the degree of a congenital colour defect, measure colour vision binocularly. If you are assessing acquired colour defects, measure monocularly.
4. Seat the patient comfortably at a table wearing his or her habitual near vision correction.
5. Hold the test in your hand or place it on the table in front of the patient, about 35 cm away with the pages at right angles to the patient's line of sight. The cap colours can become soiled with time and some practitioners use white cotton gloves (photographer's) for themselves and the patient.
6. Show the demonstration plate A to the patient and describe the test: "Here are four coloured spots surrounding one in the middle. Please tell me which of the four spots is nearest in *colour* to the one in the middle. Either point or tell me whether it is the top, bottom, left or right, but please don't touch the pages."
7. Show the test plates 1 to 10 in turn. Allow about 3 sec per page, with a slightly longer time for the first few pages while the patient becomes familiar with the task.
8. Record the patient's choices in the appropriate column on the record card (either RE, LE or both).

Recording. The TCU record form (Figure 2.4) indicates the most likely of the four spots which will be called as most similar to the middle by colour normals, protans, deutans and tritans. This can be used to categorise a colour defect in a patient who makes some mistakes. Score the patient's responses out of 10. The number of mistakes in the normal column indicates the severity of the colour defect. Record if the patient was unusually slow.

Interpretation. A patient 'fails' the test if they make more than two mistakes. A patient who makes one or two mistakes is 'borderline' and may require retesting or testing with a more extensive battery of tests. The TCU grades the severity and classifies the colour deficiency. Patients who fail the Ishihara and then pass the TCU have a mild red–green defect, and are unlikely to have trouble with most occupations.

City University colour vision test

Address .... Patient ....

Examiner .... Male/Female Date .... / .... /199 ....

Spectacles worn? Yes/No   RE/LE/BE

Illumination ('Daylight')   Type .... Level ....

FORMULA: Here are four colour spots surrounding one in the centre. Tell me which spot
looks most near in *colour* to the one in the centre. Use the words 'TOP',
'BOTTOM', 'RIGHT' or 'LEFT'. Please do not touch the pages.

Page (A is for demonstration	Subject's choice of match R I L IBoth	Normal	Diagnosis		
			Protan	Deutan	Tritan
1		B ⬇	R	L	T
2		R ➡	B	L	T
3		L ⬅	R	T	B
4		R ➡	L	B	T
5		L ⬅	T	B	R
6		B ⬇	L	T	R
7		L ⬅	T	R	B
8		R ➡	L	B	T
9		B ⬇	L	T	R
10		T ⬆	B	L	R

'Chroma four' — pages 1–6
'Chroma two' — pages 7–10

SCORE	At chroma four	/6	/6	/6	/6
	At chroma two	/4	/4	/4	/4
	Overall	/10	/10	/10	/10

Probable type   P; PA, EPA mixed
of Daltonism   D, DA, EDA
                  Tritan

Figure 2.4 The record form of The City University colour vision test (TCU). Reproduced
with permission from Keeler Ltd.

Most common errors
1. Using an unsuitable light source.
2. Allowing the patient too long to look at the figures.
3. Suggesting to the patient which spot might be correct.

Further reading

Adams, A.J. and Haegerstrom-Portnoy, G. (1987). Colour deficiency. In *Diagnosis and Management of Vision Care* (J.F. Amos, ed.) Butterworth–Heinemann, Oxford, UK
Birch, J. (1993). *Diagnosis of Defective Colour Vision*. Oxford University Press, Oxford, UK

Anterior curvature of the cornea

Background

Measurement of the anterior curvature of the cornea, called keratometry, is useful in both contact lenses fitting and their after-care. In contact lens fitting, keratometer measurements are used to indicate the corneal shape and thus the contact lens shape which might be an appropriate fit and which could be tried first. In contact lens after-care, keratometer readings can be used to monitor lens-induced corneal surface changes. For example, distortion of the keratometer mires can indicate unwanted mechanical action of the lens on the cornea, and a steepening cornea can indicate oedema.

The keratometer can also be used to measure the base curve of rigid contact lenses, and provide an indication of tear film quality. Tear break-up time can be measured as the number of seconds between a blink and the first indication of distortion of the mire images.

Apart from contact lens work, the keratometer can be used as an aid in the diagnosis of ocular pathology. The keratometer mire images (see Figures 2.5 and 2.6) would typically be distorted in cases of corneal disease such as keratoconus, corneal scarring, lid neoplasms, chalazia or pterygia, or other conditions which could cause mechanical stretching or compression of the corneal surface. Keratometry is therefore mandatory in contact lens work and optional, as an aid to diagnosis, in some ocular pathologies.

Recommended test: One position (Bausch and Lomb type) or two position variable doubling keratometer

Rationale

Both these instruments (or copies of) are in widespread use in optometric practice. The one position instrument is said to be quicker to use since once aligned on one of the corneal principal meridians, both principal meridians can be measured without further adjustment, hence the 'one position' name.

Disadvantages include that the instrument design assumes that the principal meridians lie exactly at 90 degrees to each other, which is not always the case, especially when the cornea has been subjected to contact lens wear. Also, as it is a one position instrument, both the vertical and horizontal mires are imaged at the same time and in higher degrees of corneal toricity, this can mean the vertical mire is not in focus at the same focusing position as the horizontal mire. Lastly, the Bausch and Lomb keratometer tends to use a shorter working distance than two position instruments and this can lead to larger measurement errors. Of course, if either of the two mentioned situations are encountered, the keratometer can be turned to the second principal meridian and the second reading taken in a 'two position' style.

Two position variable mire keratometers include the Javal Schiotz and copies. Measurements of corneal radii are achieved by the physical movement of the mires along an arc. The main criticism of this instrument is that unlike the variable doubling keratometer, where measurements are made on a linear scale, radii which fall at the extreme ends of the arc are non-linear and this can lead to measurement inaccuracy.

Perhaps the best instrument is the two position variable doubling keratometer, especially if it is of telecentric design. The advantage of telecentricity is that focusing of the eyepiece of the telescope is not necessary and therefore there are no inaccuracies due to focusing errors. Unfortunately these telecentric instruments can be expensive and are not commonly encountered. Although two position variable doubling instruments do require a second adjustment of the instrument to find and measure the second principal meridian, they tend to be more accurate because of a longer working distance.

Newer and more complex instruments are being marketed which potentially give more information about the corneal surface. Autokeratometers, for example, measure both central and peripheral corneal radii. The EyeSys and TMS instruments are more complex still and use 16 mire images in the form of concentric circles with readings taken along 256 corneal meridians. The topography of the cornea can therefore be mapped with these instruments. The current cost of such equipment probably precludes common adoption except perhaps in the busiest and most wide-ranging contact lens practice.

Since one and two position instruments are the most commonly encountered, the measurement procedures for these particular instruments are outlined below.

Procedure for the Bausch and Lomb one position keratometer

1. Seat the patient comfortably in front of the keratometer, and ask him or her to remove any glasses. Sit opposite the patient, across the instrument table, and dim the room lighting.
2. Explain to the patient that you are going to measure the shape of the front of the eye/cornea so that you will know which contact lens to fit, or so that you can tell if the contact lens is changing the shape of the cornea.
3. Adjust the eyepiece of the instrument by turning the eyepiece anticlockwise as far as it will go. Place a white sheet of paper in front of the telescope part of the instrument and turn the eyepiece clockwise until the black cross hair just comes into sharp focus.
4. Adjust the height of the patient's chair and the instrument to a comfortable position for both you and the patient. Ask the patient to lean forward and place his or her chin in the chin rest and forehead against the head rest. Occlude the eye not being tested by swinging the instrument's occluder into place. Then adjust the chin rest so that the outer canthus aligns with the head rest marker.
5. Ask the patient to look at the image of his or her own eye in the centre of the instrument and to open the eye wide after a full blink. If a high refractive error prevents the patient seeing his or her own eye, then ask the patient to look into the centre of the instrument. Make vertical adjustments of the instrument if the patient is unable to see into the centre.
6. Align the instrument so that the lower right mire image is in the centre of the crosshairs, and lock the instrument into place.
7. Adjust the focusing of the instrument by turning the focusing knob until the telescope is at its maximum distance away from the patient. This means that to focus the mire images requires you to move the telescope towards the patient. Focus the instrument until the mires are clear and the lower right mire is no longer doubled.
8. If you cannot focus the mires, check to see that the patient's head is firmly against the head rest. If the patient is in the correct position, and the mires are still out of focus, adjust the position of the head rest

forward or backward while continuing to focus until the mires are in focus.

9. Measure the principal meridian which is closest to the horizontal first. Use one hand to adjust the focusing knob to ensure a single, clear mire image, and adjust the horizontal alignment wheel to superimpose the two plus signs with the other hand (Figure 2.5).
10. Measure the second principal meridian which is theoretically 90° to the primary one. Adjust the focusing knob and the vertical alignment wheel until the minus signs are superimposed (Figure 2.5).
11. Rotate the instrument so that the plus signs are exactly superimposed on each other. This ensures that the instrument is aligned precisely on a principal meridian.
12. Make any further adjustments necessary to exactly superimpose the mires.

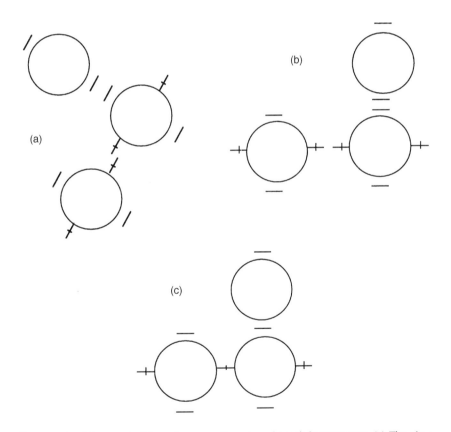

Figure 2.5 Alignment of the mires on a Bausch and Lomb keratometer. (a) The view when the mires are off the principal meridians. (b) The view when the mires are on the principal meridians. (c) The view when the plus and minus signs are overlapping to measure the 'horizontal' and 'vertical' radii of curvature.

13. Note the radii of the principal meridians in millimetres and the direction of the meridians in degrees. Most instruments also have a dioptric scale and this may be recorded also.
14. Repeat the measurements on the other eye.

Procedure for two position variable doubling type keratometer

1. Set up the patient and the instrument as described in steps 1–8 above.
2. Move the telescope forward by adjusting the focusing knob appropriately. You may need to make minor adjustments both horizontally and vertically to centre the mire images and achieve a view as depicted in Figure 2.6. If the blocks and staircase are on the same level (Figure 2.6a), then the angle of the instrument arc is aligned with a principal meridian of the cornea and you can proceed to step 4.
3. If the picture you see is similar to Figure 2.6c, where the blocks and staircase are not on the same level, then the angle of the instrument arc is not aligned along a principal meridian. Move the arc slowly until the staircase and block mires are on the same level and are able to be brought into contact, as in Figure 2.6d, by turning the knurled knob situated below the arc.
4. Ask the patient to blink and then keep the eyes as wide open as possible. Turn the knurled knob situated below the arc until the staircase and block mires are just touching. If you turn the knob too much and the mires overlap, a white area of overlap will be seen. Adjust the position of the mires until they are just touching with no overlap. If the hair wire does not cross through the middle of

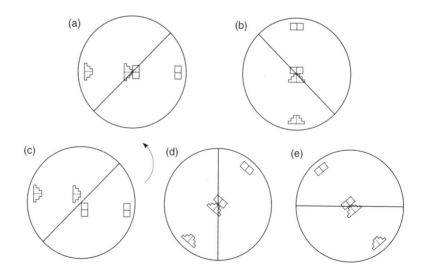

Figure 2.6 The mire images as seen on the Javal Schiotz keratometer. (a) Aligned mire images along the horizontal. (b) Mires from (a) touching with no overlap. (c) Non-aligned mire images. (d) Mire images from (c) brought into alignment along an oblique meridian. (e) Mires from (d) touching with no overlap.

the touching mires, make final horizontal and vertical adjustments to achieve this.

5. Read off the angle of the arc from the degree scale of the instrument and the radius of curvature along this meridian from the millimetre scale.

6. Turn the arc through 90° and make adjustments as in steps 4 and 5 to achieve a picture similar to Figures 2.6b or 2.6e. Note the reading off the scales. This is the corneal radius along the other meridian.

Recording

The results are recorded with the horizontal meridian first followed by the vertical as follows:

R 7.75 @ 175, 7.60 @ 85

L 7.70 @ 180, 7.60 @ 90

The @ nomenclature can be replaced by 'along'. A degree sign (°) should not be used after the axis direction. It is possible for the degree symbol to be confused with a zero, so that 15 degrees could become 150 degrees.

Interpretation

A small radius means a steep corneal surface, whereas larger radii mean flatter surfaces. Corneal astigmatism is usually less than 2.00 D and the radius of curvature is normally between 8.50 mm and 7.25 mm. It is most common to find the flattest corneal meridian lying along the horizontal (with-the-rule astigmatism) in younger patients. Little change in curvature occurs between the mid-teens and the late forties. Over the age of 40, there is a significant shift towards against-the-rule astigmatism. Unusually steep readings with irregular principal meridians are indicative of keratoconus. Large changes in the degree of astigmatism within a short time can be indicative of lid neoplasms, chalazia or a hordeolum.

The corneal astigmatism is called oblique when the principle meridians are between 30° and 60° and 120° and 150°. You should make a note of any irregularities in the mires as viewed through the keratometer. Note that the repeatability of keratometer measurements is such that accuracy to greater than 0.05 mm is not possible, and you should not interpolate between 0.05 mm scale divisions.

Most common errors

1. Not making sure the patient keeps his or her head against the head rest.
2. Forgetting to focus the eyepieces.
3. Not centring the mire images.
4. Not getting the patient to fixate properly.
5. Not determining the correct axis.
6. Forgetting to calibrate the instrument on a regular basis; this should be carried out using a steel ball (usually 7.95 mm radius of curvature).

The ball is placed on a mount or clamp, or on the side of the head rest at eye level, using plasticine. The instrument should be aligned and focused in the normal way. Any deviation from 7.95 mm means that you should re-calibrate the instrument according to the equipment manual.

Further reading

Douthwaite, W.A. (1995). *Contact Lens Optics and Design*. Butterworth–Heinemann, Oxford, UK
Stockwell, H. and Stone, J. (1988). Anterior Eye Examination. In *Optometry* (K. Edwards and R. Llewellyn, eds) Butterworth–Heinemann, Oxford, UK

Measurement of interpupillary distance (PD)

Background

The distance between the entrance pupils of the eyes is measured for two reasons: (1) to place the optical centre of the trial frame/phoropter lens(es) in front of the patient's visual axis to control prism and to avoid aberrations; and (2) so that the optical centre of spectacle lenses can be placed in front of the patient's visual axis to avoid unwanted prism and aberrations, or deliberately placed elsewhere to produce desired prism.

Recommended test: Direct measurement using a PD ruler

Rationale

This technique is quick and convenient to use during an examination as it requires no instrumentation other than a simple millimetre ruler. Direct measurement for binocular PD is about as accurate with a PD ruler as it is using a pupillometer. A pupillometer should be used for monocular measurements, such as when dispensing varifocal or high powered lenses.

Procedure

1. Keep the room lights on.
2. Explain to the patient that you are going to measure the distance between his or her eyes so that you can put any lenses in the correct position for their eyes.
3. Face the patient directly at the distance desired for the near PD (usually about 40 cm).
4. Rest the PD ruler on the bridge of the patient's nose or on the forehead so that the millimetre scale is within the spectacle plane. Steady your hand with your fingers on the patient's temple to ensure that the ruler is held firmly in place.
5. Close your right eye and ask the patient to look at your left eye. (It is usually easiest to indicate with your finger the eye that you want the patient to fixate.)
6. Choose a point of reference on the patient's right eye. The temporal pupil margin is usually most convenient, although the centre of the pupil or the temporal limbus margin may also be used and the latter may be essential with patients with dark irides. Align the zero point on the ruler with this reference point.

7. Sighting with your left eye only, look over to the patient's left eye and note the reading on the ruler that aligns with the corresponding reference point on the left eye. This would be the left nasal pupil margin if you used the temporal pupil margin of the right eye. This reading represents the near interpupillary distance since the patient will be converging to fixate your open eye binocularly. Normally this is done at 40 cm but, if desired, the near PD can be measured for a closer or farther working distance simply by decreasing or increasing the distance between the examiner's eye and the patient's eye. The closer the near PD is measured, the smaller it will be due to the increased convergence demand.

8. To measure the distance PD, first ensure that the zero point on the PD ruler is still aligned with the patient's right eye reference point using your left eye. Next close your left eye, open your right and ask the patient to change fixation to your open right eye. Take care not to move the ruler or your head position. By sighting again to the appropriate reference point on the patient's left eye, you will obtain a reading for the distance PD (see Figure 2.7).

Recording

The values are normally recorded as distance PD/near PD (in mm), for example 63/60.

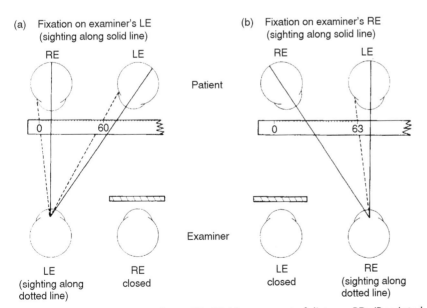

Figure 2.7 (a) Measurement of near PD. (b) Measurement of distance PD. (Reprinted with permission from Hrynchak, P. (1996). *Procedures in Clinical Optometry*. University of Waterloo Press, Waterloo, Canada.)

Interpretation

For women the distance PD is most commonly in the range of 55 to 65 mm, and for men, 59 to 70 mm. Young children may have PDs as low as 45 mm. The distance PD value is usually 3 or 4 mm greater than the near PD at 40 cm.

When adjusting a phoropter or trial frame for distance testing, the lenses are placed such that the distance between their optical centres equals the patient's distance PD. This is also true when prescribing spectacle lenses for distance viewing. Similarly, when near testing is performed or spectacles are prescribed for near work, the lenses are normally centred at the near PD. In certain cases, the optical centres of spectacle lenses are decentred from the PD so that a specific magnitude of lateral or vertical prism is introduced.

Most common errors

1. Moving the ruler during the measurement. Make sure it is held firmly and steadily in position. After taking the distance PD reading, it is a good idea to re-open your left eye, have the patient switch fixation back to it and check that the zero mark on the ruler is still aligned with the original reference point on the patient's right eye.
2. Using an inaccurate near test distance, most commonly unwittingly drifting in closer than 40 cm so the near PD turns out to be lower than it should be. The test distance should not affect the distance PD measurement.

3
Refraction

Objective measurement of refractive error

Background

An objective measurement of refractive error is the only assessment available in patients who are unable to co-operate in a subjective refraction, such as young children and the developmentally delayed. It is also heavily relied upon when subjective responses are limited (non English-speaking patients and patients whose subjective responses are poor, including some low vision patients) or unreliable (malingerers and patients with ocular hysteria). In more routine patients, it provides an objective first measure of refractive error which can be refined by subjective refraction.

Recommended test: Retinoscopy

Procedure

1. Seat the patient comfortably in the examining chair. Set the patient's distance PD in the trial frame or phoropter. Position the trial frame or phoropter before the patient so that the lenses will be in the patient's spectacle plane (approximately 12 mm from the cornea). Make sure that the trial frame or phoropter is level.

2. Either

   (a) Place working distance lenses in the back cells of the trial frame (+2.00 DS for a 50 cm working distance, +1.50 DS for 67 cm). Most phoropters contain a built-in +1.50 DS ret. lens which can be used. This technique has the advantage that all 'with' movements indicate hyperopia and all 'against' movements indicate myopia. It also provides a 'fogging' lens which will relax any low hyperopia

or

   (b) Do not add a working distance lens. The working distance power (+1.50 D or +2.00 D usually) must later be subtracted from your final retinoscope result. This technique has the advantages that you avoid introducing two reflection surfaces from the working distance lens which can make retinoscopy easier, and it frees up a trial frame cell.

Rationale

Autorefraction is a useful and reliable alternative to retinoscopy in some patients. However, autorefractor results can be unreliable or unobtainable in patients with high refractive errors, small pupils, media opacities and pseudophakia. Some studies have found results can be more minus (or less plus) than subjective refraction in young patients due to proximal or instrument accommodation. Autorefraction does not provide the sensitive assessment of the ocular media that retinoscopy does provide (e.g. early detection of cataracts, keratoconus). Auto-refraction is also more expensive and non-portable.

There is little to choose between using streak or spot retinoscopes or negative and positive cylinders. The procedure is described for streak retinoscopy, but spot retinoscopy is an acceptable alternative. Positive cylinders have the advantage of making retinoscopy easier to learn. However, negative cylinders are preferred as they are found in most phoropters. In addition, there is the possibility of stimulating accommodation during subjective refraction when removing a plus cylinder from the trial frame to replace it with one of another power.

3. Switch on the duochrome and switch the room lights off. You may wish to use the anglepoise lamp to light up the trial case.

4. Explain the test to the patient: "I'm going to shine a light in your eye and get an indication of the power of the glasses you will need. Please look at the red and green target in the mirror, and let me know if my head blocks your view. Do not worry if the chart is blurred".

5. Sit or stand off to the side of the patient so that manipulation of the trial frame/phoropter is easy. Use a comfortable working distance from the patient so that you can change lenses in the spectacle plane easily (a comfortable arm's length is often 67 cm or 50 cm). You should be on the patient's right side and use your right hand and right eye to check the patient's right eye and vice versa for the left eye.

6. Set the retinoscope mirror to the plano position (maximum divergence) and position the retinoscope so that you are looking along the visual axis of the patient's eye (the patient's other eye is fixating the duochrome). As he or she will generally look slightly upwards to view the duochrome, to look along the patient's visual axis you will need to be slightly higher than the patient.

7. Initially, rotate the retinoscope about an axis parallel to your facial plane and perpendicular to the floor while looking through the aperture. This will cause the reflex to move in the pupil. If the reflex moves in the same direction as the movement of the retinoscopic streak, this is known as 'with' movement. If the reflex moves in the opposite direction as the movement of the retinoscopic streak, this is known as 'against' movement. Rotate the retinoscopic streak, using the controls on the retinoscope, through 180° and observe the differences in the speed and width of the reflex movement in all meridians.

8. If the patient is pre-presbyopic and a hyperope, it is advisable to place positive lenses before both eyes to ensure that accommodation is as relaxed as possible and an accurate ret. result can be obtained. If you are using working distance lenses, this is only necessary for moderate hyperopes (above +1.50 or +2.00 DS).

9. If the reflex is very dim or hard to interpret, the patient either has media opacities or small pupils or is a high hyperope or high myope. Move increasingly closer to the patient's eye as this can make the movement of the reflex easier to see. If there is now a slow 'with' or 'against' movement, the patient is a high ametrope, so add an appropriate medium-to-large powered lens and repeat retinoscopy at the normal distance.

10. With no lenses in place, determine if the refractive error is spherical (the observed reflex has the same speed, direction and thickness in all meridians) or astigmatic (the reflex differs in different meridians). If the reflex movement is relatively slow and any difference between the reflex speed and thickness is difficult to determine, place an appropriate lens in the trial frame to get nearer to neutrality, and check again for astigmatism (Figure 3.1).

11. If astigmatic, determine the principal meridians by rotating the streak axis until the angle of the reflex movement coincides with the angle of the streak in two meridians; one perpendicular to the other (see

Figure 3.1). If the principal meridians are hard to pinpoint, adjust the mirror position slightly to narrow the streak width.

12. Determine the spherical component by 'neutralising' (adding plus lenses to 'with' movement and minus lenses to 'against' movement until the reflex fills the entire pupil and all perceived movement stops) the most plus/least minus meridian first (plano mirror: fastest 'against' or slowest 'with'). To neutralise a given meridian, the streak is oriented perpendicular to that meridian and moved along that meridian (e.g. to neutralise the vertical meridian, the streak is horizontal and moves vertically). If the cylinder amount is small and the most plus/least minus meridian is difficult to determine, then neutralise one meridian and then check the other. If the most plus/least minus meridian was neutralised first, then the second meridian should be showing 'against' motion for the plano mirror position. Use a bracketing technique to determine neutrality. The neutral point can be checked by moving backward and forward slightly and checking the movement of the reflex. A 'with' movement should be seen when you move forward, and an 'against' movement when you move backward.

13. Set the minus cylinder axis parallel with the streak orientation of the least plus/most minus meridian. Position the retinoscope streak along this meridian and you should observe 'against' movement. Add minus cylinder in a bracketing technique to achieve neutrality. As 'with' movement can be easier to see than 'against' movement, you may wish to add minus cylinder until 'with' movement is just seen and then reduce the cylinder by 0.25 D. Alternatively, you may wish to neutralise the cylinder with the retinoscope in the concave mirror position, in which case you will add minus cylinder to neutralise 'with' movement.

14. Briefly, recheck the sphere and cylinder components for neutrality.

15. Repeat steps 3 to 10 on the patient's left eye.

16. Recheck the right eye. This step may not be necessary if you have ensured that no accommodation has taken place throughout the procedure (see step 8). Recheck the left eye if the right eye is changed.

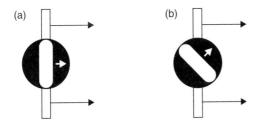

Figure 3.1 Determining the two astigmatic meridians. (a) If you are 'retting' on axis, the reflex will move in the same direction as the retinoscopy streak. (b) If you are off axis, the reflex will move in a different direction from the direction of the retinoscopy streak. You should then rotate your streak to align with the reflex.

17. Remove the +1.50 (or +2.00) working distance lenses (or subtract 1.50 or 2.00 D from your final result).
18. Measure the patient's visual acuities with the net retinoscope result.

Recording

Record the sphero-cylinder correction that neutralised the patient's refractive error after removing your working distance lenses, and the visual acuities with those lenses, e.g.

$$-2.00/-1.00 \times 35; +4.25/-0.75 \times 95$$

Do not include DS (dioptres of spherical power), DC (dioptres of cylindrical power) or a degree sign in this recording of the sphere–cylinder correction. Use 'x' rather than the word axis. Record the spherical power to the nearest 0.25 D, and the cylinder axis to the nearest 2.5 degrees. The axis should be between 2.5 degrees and 180 degrees. Use 180 rather than 0 degrees.

Interpretation

The following classification of refractive error is commonly used:

1. Simple myopia: minus sphere lens only.
2. Simple hyperopia: plus sphere lens only.
3. Simple myopic astigmatism: plano sphere with minus cylinder.
4. Simple hyperopic astigmatism: plus sphere of same power as minus cylinder.
5. Compound myopic astigmatism: minus sphere with minus cylinder.
6. Compound hyperopic astigmatism: plus sphere with minus cylinder of less magnitude than the sphere.
7. Mixed astigmatism: plus sphere with minus cylinder of greater magnitude than the sphere.

Latent hyperopes can show much more plus in retinoscopy than they will accept in a dry (non-cycloplegic) refraction. Patients with media opacities and/or small pupils may have dim reflexes which make retinoscopy difficult. In this situation, you may be able to obtain a better reflex by performing retinoscopy at a reduced working distance of say 25 or 33 cm. Do not use a working distance lens and use as small a number of lenses as possible with these patients as you will lose 8% of the reflex for each lens used due to reflections. You will have to subtract a larger value from your ret. result to compensate for the reduced working distance (4.00 or 3.00 D respectively for the two distances mentioned above).

Most common errors

1. Performing retinoscopy off-axis.
2. Performing retinoscopy at an incorrect working distance, e.g. working at about 50 cm, while using a 1.50 D working distance lens.

3. Blocking the patient's view of the distance chart, thereby likely stimulating accommodation.
4. Confusing the retinoscope collar positions.
5. Holding the lenses away from the spectacle plane.
6. Not concentrating on the movement in the centre of the pupil only in a patient with large pupils.

Acceptable alternative procedure: Spot retinoscopy

As the name suggests, spot retinoscopy uses a spot of light rather than a streak. Therefore there is no need to rotate the streak to determine the astigmatic meridians. In an astigmatic eye, the spot retinoscopic reflex is elliptical rather than circular, and the two astigmatic meridians are determined by the long and short axes of the ellipse. Otherwise the procedure is the same as for streak retinoscopy.

Further reading

Bennett, A.G. and Rabbetts, R.B. (1993). *Clinical Visual Optics*. Butterworth–Heinemann, Oxford, UK
Mutti, D. O. and Zadnik, K. (1997) Refractive error. In *The Ocular Examination: Measurements and Findings* (K. Zadnik, ed.) W.B. Saunders, London, UK.

Subjective refraction

Background

The examiner communicates with the patient and, using the patient's responses to the vision through various lenses, determines the optical correction which best suits the patient.

Recommended tests

For beginning students, monocular refraction followed by binocular balancing is recommended. For students in later years and practitioners, the modified Humphriss immediate contrast refraction (binocular refraction) procedure is recommended.

Rationale
As most patients view the world binocularly, it seems appropriate to measure the refractive error under binocular conditions. Binocular refraction has several advantages over monocular refraction, the main one being that there is better control over, and greater relaxation of, accommodation. This is particularly important when measuring the refractive error in patients with hyperopia, pseudomyopia and antimetropia. Binocular refraction is also preferred in patients with latent nystagmus and any cyclo-

deviation. The occluder used in monocular refraction manifests latent nystagmus and makes subjective refraction difficult. The occluder can also manifest any cyclophoria which could lead to an incorrect assessment of astigmatism. Finally, binocular refraction has the advantage of being slightly quicker than monocular refraction in that no binocular balancing is required. The Humphriss immediate contrast refraction method is recommended as it is simple to perform and requires no extra equipment. Other binocular refraction methods include using a septum or polarisation techniques.

Monocular refraction followed by binocular balancing

Procedure

1. The subjective refraction generally follows retinoscopy. If not, set the patient's distance PD in the trial frame or phoropter. Position the trial frame or phoropter before the patient so that the lenses will be in the patient's spectacle plane (approximately 12 mm from the cornea). Make sure that the trial frame or phoropter is level.
2. Sit or stand off to the side of the patient so that manipulation of the trial frame/phoropter is easy.
3. Begin with the net retinoscopy sphere–cylinder before each eye.
4. The subjective refraction traditionally begins on the right eye (or the poorer eye if you determine there may be a poor eye from the case Hx). Occlude the left eye.
5. Determine the best sphere:

    (a) Direct the patient's attention to the best acuity line of the right eye. Add +0.25 D and ask: "Are the letters clearer, more blurred or the same?"

      (i) If the acuity improves or *remains the same* with the additional plus, then continue adding +0.25 DS until the acuity first blurs. Stop at the most plus/least minus lens that does not blur the visual acuity.
      (ii) If the visual acuity blurs with a +0.25 DS lens, then do not add it.

    (b) Add a −0.25 D lens. If visual acuity improves with the lens, then add further minus lenses (in 0.25 D steps) *only as long as the visual acuity improves*. If the young patient (with accommodation) reports that vision is improved with the lens, but there is no improvement in visual acuity, ask whether the letters definitely look clearer or just smaller and blacker. If the letters just look smaller and blacker, do not add the −0.25 DS. If the patient reports no change or a worsening of vision, do not add the +0.25 DS.

6. Duochrome check. Check that the rings on the duochrome look equally clear and black on the red and green, indicating that the best mean sphere has been obtained and the circle of least confusion is on the retina. If the rings on the green look clearer, add +0.25 DS until you obtain a balance. If the rings on the red look clearer, add

−0.25 DS until you obtain a balance. If you cannot balance the duochrome, leave the rings on the green slightly clearer, as younger patients with accommodation will then be able to bring the circle of least confusion onto the retina.

7. Check test for cylinder axis. Note that the plus cylinder axis is in red on the hand-held Jackson cross cylinder (X-cyl) with the minus axis in white. On phoropters, the reverse is true.

   (a) Illuminate the concentric rings or indicate a circular letter one or two rows above the present visual acuity. Move the X-cyl in front of the trial frame/phoropter aperture.

   (b) Instruct the patient: "I am going to show you two pictures of the *. Both pictures may be slightly blurred, but I want you to tell me which is the clearer of the two pictures, or whether they look the same".

   (c) If cylinder was found with retinoscopy, proceed with step 7(e).

   (d) If there has been no cylinder found with retinoscopy, then set the X-cyl so that its minus cylinder axis and the perpendicular plus cylinder axis assume the 90° and 180° positions. It does not matter which dot is at 90° and 180°. Refer to the current X-cyl orientation as 'lens or picture 1'. Flip the X-cyl to reverse the positions of the minus and plus axes. Refer to this latter orientation as 'lens or picture 2'. Note the orientation of the minus cylinder axis in the position in which the patient reported that vision was best. Rotate the X-cyl so that the plus and minus cylinder axes assume the 45° and 135° positions. Repeat the above comparison and note the orientation of the minus cylinder axis of the chosen lens. If all the lenses seem equally clear, then there is no cylinder and you should proceed to step 9. If certain lens positions are preferred, then set the phoropter cylinder axis at or between the indicated axes (e.g. if minus cylinder was called for at 180° and 45°, then set the phoropter cylinder axis to the approximate midpoint, i.e. 25°). Place −0.25 or −0.50 D cylinder power in the phoropter and proceed with the next step. If you add −0.50 DC, add +0.25 DS to the spherical lens to keep the circle of least confusion on the retina.

   (e) Set the X-cyl so that the minus cylinder axis and the plus cylinder axis straddle the trial frame/phoropter cylinder axis (Figure 3.2). With most phoropters the X-cyl will click into place at this correct orientation. Have the patient compare this initial lens position 'lens 1' to its flipped counterpart 'lens 2' (Figure 3.2).

   (f) Adjust the X-cyl and trial frame/phoropter cylinder axes about 5° (it may be appropriate to use larger steps for low cylinder powers) toward the minus cylinder axis of the preferred lens position (1 or 2). Repeat the comparison and adjust the axis until the patient notices no difference between the two lens positions (or until the examiner has bracketed the axis). If the

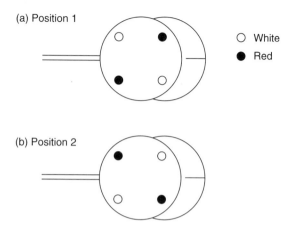

(a) Position 1

○ White
● Red

(b) Position 2

Figure 3.2 Orientation of the cross cylinder for axis determination in (a) 'picture or lens 1' and (b) 'picture or lens 2'.

two lenses appear equally blurred to the patient, then move on to step 7(g).

(g) If the two initial lens positions appear the same, confirm that the current axis is the correct one by moving the trial frame/phoropter cylinder axes off by about 5° (use larger steps for low cylinder powers) and having the patient compare lens 1 and 2. The patient should return you to the initial axis orientation if it was correct. If the patient does not, he or she may be a relatively poor observer and have a range of cylinder axes positions in which the X-cyl positions look the same. In this case, you need to determine the extent of this range and place the cylinder axis in the middle of it (e.g. if the patient reports that the X-cyl positions look the same at 20° through to 40°, place the cylinder axis at 30°. You could also use a ±0.50 X-cyl with such patients).

8. Check test for cylinder power. Note that the plus cylinder axis is in red on the hand-held X-cyl with the minus axis in white. On phoropters, the reverse is true.

   (a) Orient the X-cyl so that either the minus axis or plus axis parallels the trial frame/phoropter cylinder axis (the X-cyl should click into place with most phoropters). Have the patient compare the relative clarity of lens 1 to lens 2 as before (Figure 3.3).

   (b) If there is no difference between lens 1 and 2, then remove a −0.25 D cylinder and repeat the comparison. If the initial lens was correct, the patient will call for more cylinder by choosing the lens that has the minus cylinder axis parallel to the phoropter axis. In this case, increase the cylinder power to its original amount.

   (c) If there is a difference between lens 1 and 2, then add minus cylinder (−0.25 D) if the patient prefers the minus cylinder axis

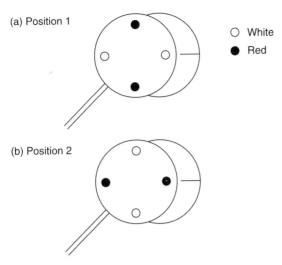

(a) Position 1

○ White
● Red

(b) Position 2

Figure 3.3 Orientation of the cross cylinder for power determination in (a) 'picture or lens 1' and (b) 'picture or lens 2'.

parallel to the phoropter axis. Remove −0.25 DC if the patient prefers the plus cylinder axis parallel to the phoropter axis. Continue this process until no difference between lens 1 and 2 can be detected or until the power has been bracketed to less than 0.25 D (choose the least minus cylinder).

(d) For each 0.50 D change in cylinder power, change the sphere power by 0.25 D in the opposite direction (e.g. if you add −0.50 D of cylinder, then add +0.25 D of sphere before comparing the lens positions). This is to ensure that the circle of least confusion remains on the retina.

9. Accommodation checks, such as the duochrome or +1.00 test should now be performed:

(a) The +1.00 DS check. With the fellow eye occluded, visual acuity should drop about four lines when a +1.00 DS is placed over the final refraction. Visual acuity should drop to 6/12 or 6/18 in a patient with 6/5 with the final Rx. If the visual acuity only drops to 6/6 or 6/9, then it is likely that the subjective refraction is overminused (or underplussed) and should be rechecked

and/or

(b) Duochrome check. The patient is asked which rings on the duochrome look clearer and blacker, on the red or the green. The rings should look about the same or the rings on the red could appear slightly clearer. With a −0.25 DS, the rings on the green background should become slightly clearer and blacker. If the rings on the green are clearer and blacker to begin with, then this suggests that the subjective refraction is overminused (or underplussed) and should be rechecked.

10. Measure visual acuity.
11. Repeat steps 4–9 for the other eye.
12. If your patient has some accommodation left (i.e. they are younger than about 55 years), you will now perform a binocular balance of accommodation. You can use a modified Humphriss binocular balance or a Turville infinity balance (see later). The Humphriss binocular balance method is as follows:

    (a) Fog the left eye until the visual acuity is reduced by 3 or 4 lines less than the tested eye. Young patients with normal vision would usually require adding +0.75 DS or +1.00 DS to give a visual acuity of about 6/12. For older patients, +1.00 DS or +1.25 DS may be required, as dioptric blur has less of an effect due to the smaller pupil in older patients.
    (b) Repeat the assessment of the best mean sphere as described in step 5 above.

13. Binocular add check. Place +0.25 DS in front of both eyes, and ask if the letters become clearer, more blurred or are unchanged. As before, if the acuity improves or remains the same with the additional plus, then continue adding +0.25 DS binocularly until the acuity first blurs. Stop at the most plus/least minus lens that does not blur the visual acuity. If the binocular visual acuity blurs with the +0.25 DS lenses, then do not add them.

    Then add −0.25 D lenses binocularly. If the visual acuity is unchanged or decreased, then do not add the lens. If visual acuity improves with the lens, then add further minus lenses binocularly (in 0.25 D steps) *only as long as the visual acuity improves.*

Recording

Record the final monocular refraction in the format shown in the retinoscopy recording section with the corresponding visual acuities. Binocular balancing and binocular add check findings are usually recorded in a separate box on the record card. An example of a binocular balance recording could be +0.25 RE. An example of the binocular add could be +0.25. You must remember to include these when considering the final subjective refraction result.

Normal result

The subjective results should be compatible with the retinoscopy results in most cases. Inconsistent results may be due to technique error or the patient may be an unreliable observer for behavioural or visual reasons. If a patient is providing unreliable responses or is unable to tell any difference with ±0.25 DS or the ±0.25 X-cyl, then use ±0.50 DS and the ±0.50 X-cyl or even larger steps. Students generally realise that they must do this for patients with low vision as these patients cannot discriminate between the two views given with the ±0.25 X-cyl. However, this is true for any eye with reduced vision (e.g. an amblyopic eye) and also some patients with normal vision who, for whatever reason, provide poor subjective responses.

Interpretation

The difference between the patient's own spectacles and the subjective refraction should be compatible with the difference between the habitual (with own spectacles) and optimal visual acuities. For example, if the patient has a visual acuity of 6/12 in his or her spectacles and 6/5 after subjective refraction, you could expect the subjective refraction to be 1.00 DS more myopic than the spectacle Rx ($-0.25 \approx 1$ line of visual acuity). Thus, an Rx of $-1.00/-0.50 \times 180$ would become $-2.00/-0.50 \times 180$. If the subjective refraction was 1.50 to 2.00 DS more myopic, this could suggest that you have overminused the subjective refraction. Changes in hyperopic Rxs are more difficult to explain in this way as they are dependent on the amount of accommodation the patient has (and therefore their age). Changes in astigmatism are usually small.

Most common errors

1. Not monitoring the visual acuity to ensure that a change in lens power results in the expected change in visual acuity.
2. Using unclear patient instructions or leading questions.
3. Poor control of accommodation.
4. Adding minus first rather than plus first when checking the best sphere.
5. Allowing the patient to direct the examination.
6. Improper technique for checking for cylinder when no cylinder is found with retinoscopy.
7. Flipping the X-cyl lenses too fast for the patient to compare them.
8. Giving unequal presentations with the X-cyl.
9. Prescribing based only on the subjective result and not on the previous refractive and oculomotor findings.

Acceptable alternative procedures

Modified Humphriss immediate contrast refraction (binocular refraction)

Procedure. As with monocular refraction, except the whole refraction is performed under binocular conditions by first fogging rather than occluding the non-tested eye:

4. Fog the left eye until the visual acuity is reduced by three or four lines less than the tested eye. Young patients with normal vision would usually require adding +0.75 DS or +1.00 DS to give a visual acuity of about 6/12. For older patients, +1.00 DS or +1.25 DS may be required as dioptric blur has less of an effect due to the smaller pupil in older patients.

12. A binocular balance of accommodation is not required.

Advantages
1. Better control over, and greater relaxation of, accommodation. This is particularly important when measuring the refractive error in patients with hyperopia, pseudomyopia and antimetropia.
2. Preferred in patients with latent nystagmus and any cyclodeviation. The occluder used in monocular refraction manifests latent nystagmus and makes subjective refraction difficult. The occluder can also manifest any cyclophoria which could lead to an incorrect assessment of astigmatism being obtained.
3. Slightly quicker than monocular refraction as no binocular balancing is required.

Most common errors
1. Not fogging the fellow eye correctly, for example fogging by +0.75 DS when the retinoscopy result is underplussed (or overminused) significantly, so that the +0.75 DS 'fog' merely corrects the underplus of the retinoscope result rather than blurring the vision in that eye.
2. Continuing the Humphriss technique in a patient whose high dominance in the fogged eye does not allow reliable subjective responses binocularly.

For assessment of astigmatism: Fan and block

Procedure
1. Determine the best mean sphere after retinoscopy as previously explained.
2. Occlude the untested eye (i.e. LE).
3. Remove the cylinder before the right eye.
4. Determine the patient's visual acuity.
5. Add plus lenses in 0.25 D steps until the visual acuity drops by a line. Check that the circles on the duochrome are clearer and blacker on the red.
6. Draw an analogy between the lines on the fan and the hours of a clock, and ask the patient if any of the lines on the fan appear clearer and darker than the other lines.
7. Point the arrow that joins the blocks towards the clearest line. Adjust the arrow until its two arms are equally clear. One block (with its lines running parallel with those on the block which are clearest) should be clearer than the other.
8. If the patient reports that all the lines are equally clear (or blurred) then fog by a further +0.50 D and ask the patient again if any lines are clearer and darker. If they remain equally clear or blurred, then this suggests there is no astigmatism present.
9. Set the cylinder axis in the trial frame/phoropter at the axis indicated by the arrow. Add negative cylinder at this axis until the blurred block *just* becomes as clear as the other. You could start by adding the cylinder found during retinoscopy. If you cannot obtain equal clarity of the two blocks, give the lowest power cylinder.

10. Reduce the plus fogging sphere to determine the best sphere as previously explained.
11. Repeat steps 1 to 10 for the left eye.

Advantages
1. Accommodation is better controlled than with the X-cyl.
2. Can be useful in patients who provide poor responses to X-cyl.
3. Provides a fast check for the presence of astigmatism.

Disadvantages
1. May not be as accurate as X-cyl for small cylinders.
2. Not always present on some test charts.
3. Non-portable

For binocular balance of accommodation: Turville infinity balance

1. Remove the occluder from the trial frame.
2. Rotate the drum on the test chart until the F and L is shown.
3. Ask the patient to occlude the left eye and keep his or her head steady.
4. Move the septum on the mirror until it covers the L, and only the F is seen with the right eye.
5. Ask the patient to occlude the right eye now and ensure that he or she can see only the L with the left eye.
6. Ask the patient to compare, with both eyes open, the relative clarity of the F and L.
7. If the F or L are missing, recheck the position of the septum. If one is still missing, then one eye is suppressing. Any misalignment of the F and L may indicate a significant heterophoria, e.g. if the patient sees an E (F and L combined into one figure), then the patient is likely to have a high exophoria. If the F and L are misaligned vertically, then suspect a hyperphoria. These misalignments should be further investigated using appropriate tests.
8. If one of the letters is clearer than the other then perform a best mean sphere assessment (step 5 of monocular refraction above) of the eye with the least clear vision.
9. If the F and L are still not equally clear, perform a best mean sphere assessment of the other eye.

Further reading

Amos, J.F. (1991). Binocular subjective refraction. In *Clinical Procedures in Optometry* (J.B. Eskridge, J.F. Amos and J.D. Bartlett, eds) J.B. Lippincott, Philadelphia, Pennsylvania
Bennett, A.G. and Rabbetts, R.B. (eds) (1993). *Clinical Visual Optics*. Butterworth–Heinemann, Oxford, UK

Humphriss, D. (1988). Binocular refraction. In *Optometry* (K. Edwards and R. Llewellyn, eds) Butterworths, London, UK

Polasky, M. (1991). Monocular subjective refraction. In *Clinical Procedures in Optometry* (J.B. Eskridge, J.F. Amos and J.D. Bartlett, eds) J.B. Lippincott, Philadelphia, Pennsylvania

Near addition determination

Background

About the age of 40–45 years (earlier for some ethnic groups, people with short arms or working distances and hyperopes, later for people with long working distances and myopes), most people become presbyopic. This means that they do not have enough accommodation to be able to read or do other near work clearly and comfortably. These patients require a positive lens addition to the distance Rx to be able to read comfortably. This is called the reading or near addition. With increasing age and further losses in accommodation, the power of the reading addition needs to be increased. At about 55 years, accommodation is essentially zero (what can be measured clinically is probably depth of focus). After this age the reading addition still needs to be increased (perhaps to compensate for the loss of visual acuity with age), although at a slower rate.

Recommended test: Trial frame range determination

Rationale

An incorrect reading add is one of the most common causes of patient's unhappiness with his or her new spectacles. For example, patients may complain that the new spectacles are fine for reading, but that they are now unable to see their computer screen with the glasses (which they could see with their older, weaker glasses). To help to avoid such complaints, it is important to determine the range of clear near vision required by the patient and prescribe spectacles which fulfil this requirement. It is difficult to determine appropriate near working distances and ranges in a phoropter, and a trial frame add determination is recommended.

Procedure

1. The patient should remain seated in the chair with the trial frame and the balanced distance Rx in place. You should sit or stand slightly off to the patient's side but within reach of the trial frame.
2. The room lights should be on. It is often suggested that anglepoise lighting should be directed toward the reading card for determining the add. It is probably better to determine the add required in lighting conditions similar to those used regularly by the patients. Turn the anglepoise lamp on and ask them if they use similar lighting levels when performing near tasks or whether the previous room lighting was more similar. Additional lighting should be used in patients who, with their optimal near refractive correction, cannot read N5 easily without the lighting. If such patients do not have anglepoise lighting at home, they should be strongly advised to obtain some.
3. You should know from the case history what near vision tasks the patient performs. If you do not, ask for this information now. Ask the patient to hold the reading card at his or her preferred near working distance(s). Use a tape measure to determine each distance (remember a tape measure is included on the Mallett unit). For example, you may need to determine at what distances a patient sews, reads and uses a VDU.

4. If the patient's near tasks are all performed at one distance (or the patient has essentially one near vision task such as reading), then proceed to step 5. If the patient has several near vision tasks which necessitate a range of working distances (such as reading at 33 cm and using a VDU at 50 cm), proceed as follows:

(a) For younger presbyopes who retain some accommodation, determine one reading addition which allows the patient to see comfortably at all his or her required working distances. In the example above you may try to obtain a reading add which is optimal at about 40 cm (dioptrically half way between 33 and 50 cm), yet allows adequate near vision at both 33 and 50 cm. Proceed to step 5.

(b) For older presbyopes, where a single compromise add does not provide adequate near vision at one or more of the required distances, determine two (or more) reading additions, one for each of the required working distances.

(c) A combination of the above, e.g. one reading addition power may be sufficient for reading at 33 cm and sewing at 20 cm (optimally determined for 25 cm) and another power may be required for VDU use at 45 cm.

5. Tentative add determination (Table 3.1). From one or a combination of the following several rules of thumb, obtain an estimate of the reading add for the indicated working distance:

(a) By age and working distance.

(i) Patients less than 55 years of age. A quick rule of thumb for patients up to 55 years of age using an average working distance of about 40 cm is:

Tentative add = Age/10 −3.50 D

If the working distance is much less than 40 cm, increase the tentative add appropriately. If the add is needed for, e.g. VDU work and therefore the working distance is about 50–60 cm, decrease the tentative add by about +0.50 DS.

Table 3.1 Tentative reading adds at increasing ages

Age in years	Tentative add
40–45	+0.75 D
46–50	+1.25 D
51–55	+1.75 D
56–60	+2.00 D
61–65	+2.00 D
66–70	+2.25 D
70+	+2.50 D or +2.75 D

(ii) Patients over 55 years of age. After age 55 accommodation is essentially zero, and the rule given above must *not* be used. A +2.00 tentative add is a useful starting point for patients between 55 and 65 years with a working distance of about 40 cm. Again, adapt the tentative add to consider the working distance. For patients over 65 years, the reading add is determined mainly by the patient's working distance, i.e. working distances of 50, 40 or 33 cm indicate tentative adds of +2.00, +2.50 or +3.00 DS respectively.

(b) By the previous Rx and symptoms. If the previous near vision Rx was +3.00 DS for both eyes and the patient reports no problems, then an add that gives a near vision Rx of ~ +3.00 DS is a useful tentative add. If the patient reports that with this near vision Rx, he or she is having difficulty reading and it is easier if the reading material is held further away than the patient would like, then the near vision Rx is too weak and should be increased. In this case, a tentative add that gives a near vision Rx of about +3.50 DS is useful. If the patient reports that he or she has to hold near work too close to read with the present spectacles, then the Rx is too strong. In this case, a tentative add that gives a near vision Rx of about +2.50 DS is a useful tentative add.

In all these cases, you must determine how any changes in the distance Rx change the near vision Rx. Patients read through their near vision Rx (distance Rx + add), not their add, i.e. if the patient's complaints suggest that the near vision Rx is too weak ("need longer arms"; "difficulty reading"; "easier reading further away") and the distance Rx becomes more hyperopic by +0.50 DS (a typical age-related change), then the tentative add can remain the same as the old add. Because the distance Rx has increased in plus, so has the reading Rx even though the add hasn't changed!

(c) By the amplitude of accommodation. Various rules can be used to determine the tentative add from the amplitude of accommodation (e.g. reading add equals working distance in dioptres $-\frac{2}{3}$ or $\frac{1}{2}$ the amplitude of accommodation in dioptres). This is most useful for presbyopes less than 55 years of age. In older patients, their accommodation is essentially zero and age-related pupillary miosis means that any measurement of amplitude of accommodation essentially measures their depth of focus, and the rules become less useful.

(d) Tentative adds can also be determined using the cross-cylinder or plus build-up method or by balancing negative and positive relative accommodation. These methods are more commonly used by optometrists in North America and descriptions can be found in various US textbooks (see further reading).

6. Include the tentative add for each eye in the trial frame with the balanced distance Rx. Explain to the patient that you are now going to determine the power of glasses they need for near vision.

7. Adjust the trial frame for the near PD.

8. Determine the patient's monocular and binocular near visual acuity with the tentative add.

9. Determine the best add for that near working distance. Perform this test monocularly first and then binocularly.

   (a) Direct the patient's attention to the best acuity paragraph. Add -0.25 DS and ask if the letters become clearer, more blurred or are unchanged.

   (b) If the acuity improves with the additional minus, then continue adding -0.25 DS until the near acuity or clarity does not improve with the additional -0.25 D. Stop at the most minus/least plus lens that does not improve the near visual acuity or its clarity.

   (c) If the visual acuity blurs or becomes less clear with -0.25 DS lenses, then do not add them.

   (d) Add $+0.25$ DS. If the visual acuity is unchanged or decreased, then do not add the lens. If visual acuity improves with the lens, then add further minus lenses (in 0.25 D steps) only as long as the visual acuity or its clarity improves.

   (e) If the monocular values are within 0.25 DS, start with the lower add and recheck binocularly. If the monocular values are different by more than 0.25 DS, then recheck your distance correction binocular balance.

9. Determine the range of clear vision with the reading add. This is particularly important if you are intending that the reading add will be used for tasks at more than one working distance (as in step 4(a)).

   (a) To determine the near endpoint of the addition's range, have the patient move the reading card slowly in until first blur of the best acuity paragraph is reported. Measure this distance (the Mallett unit has a useful tape measure for this purpose).

   (b) Repeat this procedure to determine the far endpoint of the addition range.

   (c) Adjust the power of the add appropriately so that the range of clearest vision of the addition coincides with the near visual demands of the patient. That is, remove plus to 'place' the range of clear vision farther away from the patient and add plus to place the range closer to the patient.

10. If you are unable to obtain a range which encompasses all the near working tasks that the patient has indicated he or she performs, you will have to determine individual adds for the different working distances. For example, if you were unable to provide a good range of vision for reading (33 cm) and VDU work (50 cm) with a $+2.50$ add with best vision at 40 cm, try a $+3.00$ add at 33 cm and a $+2.00$ add at 50 cm, and repeat step 9 above for each.

11. Record the final addition(s), acuity and range of clearest vision obtained with the addition(s).

Recording

Record the tentative add and the method(s) of determination (when an undergraduate student). Record the range of near visual demands indicated by the patient. Record the final add(s), as well as the acuity attained and range of clarity for the addition.

Interpretation

Most additions are equal for the two eyes. Unequal adds require further testing; either a recheck of the balancing of the distance correction or a retest of the endpoints used for each eye. The prescribing of unequal adds between the eyes is the exception and is rarely satisfactory. Assuming no accommodative insufficiency, the power of the addition usually increases with age in patients between about 40 and 65 years old. Practitioners rarely give additions greater than +3.00 D, unless the patient's visual demands are at unusually short distances (e.g. an absolute presbyope with short arms), or are greater than the patient's visual ability (e.g. watch repairer or low vision patient). It is prudent to keep the add as weak as possible to meet the patient's need. If possible, do not change the add by more than +0.50 D to ease spectacle adaptation.

Most common errors

1. Giving extra plus when it provides no change and thus prescribing too high an addition.
2. Not determining the patient's near vision needs and subsequently prescribing an add which gives an inadequate range of clear near vision for those needs.
3. Estimating, instead of measuring, the near point distances with a tape measure.

Further reading

Fannin, T.E. (1991). Presbyopic addition. In *Clinical procedures in Optometry* (J.B. Eskridge, J.F. Amos and J.D. Bartlett, eds) J.B. Lippincott, Philadelphia, Pennsylvania
Pointer, J.S. (1995). The presbyopic add I, II & III. *Ophthal Physiol Opt*, **15**, 235–254.

4
Post-refraction binocular vision testing

Amplitude of accommodation

Background

The amplitude of accommodation represents the amount of focusing power of an eye. The amplitude of accommodation decreases with increasing age, which leads to a receding near point of clear vision. The accommodation amplitude is reduced to such an extent when people reach the age of 35–50 years that they start to have difficulty with near work. This is called presbyopia and for near work these patients require a reading addition of positive lenses to any distance correction. For these early presbyopic patients the amount of accommodation remaining can be used to indicate the power of reading add required. For older presbyopes, measuring the amplitude of accommodation is of little benefit in helping to determine the reading addition. This is because the amplitude is essentially reduced to a minimum at about 55 years of age, and what is being measured is the depth of focus. Measurement is also necessary in younger patients because a low amplitude of accommodation may result from various accommodative anomalies which can give rise to symptoms. Low accommodation for age may also be associated with systemic disease or drug side effects. Unilateral deficiency can be a sign of neurological involvement, intraocular disease or amblyopia. This test is normally performed on pre-presbyopes and early presbyopes not wearing a near reading addition.

Recommended test: Push-up amplitude of accommodation

Procedure

1. The patient should sit with the head in a normal reading position. The test is performed with the patient wearing his or her optimal distance correction. The clinician should sit directly in front of the patient to allow a clear view of both eyes simultaneously.

Rationale

The test is quick and easy to perform and gives an indication of the near range of clear vision in addition to the accommodation amplitude. It is easier to perform than using increasing amounts of minus lenses until distance vision blurs (Sheard's technique), particularly when using a trial frame.

2. Explain to the patient that you are going to measure the amount of focusing power that his or her eyes have.

3. If the test is to be performed on younger presbyopes they should wear a partial addition ($\sim$ +1.00 for 45–55 years) to ensure they can see the stimulus. In young children with very high amplitudes, slight linear differences of the near point produce large dioptric differences, and it is useful to add a $-3.00\,\mathrm{D}$ lens to place the near point further from the spectacle plane.

4. Direct the anglepoise lamp over the patient's shoulder to illuminate the print on the RAF rule.

5. The test is usually performed monocularly (right and left) followed by a measure of binocular accommodation amplitude. The procedure is common for all viewing conditions. For monocular measures occlude the appropriate eye.

6. Indicate to the patient a paragraph of N5 type on the RAF rule initially held beyond the patient's near point of accommodation. If the patient's visual acuity is less than N5, use a paragraph equal in size to the patient's resolution limit.

7. Move the target towards the patient. Instruct the patient: "Please look at the print. I am going to move it closer and I want you to tell me when it first becomes blurry". Keep moving the target until the patient notices that the letters begin to blur.

8. At this first noticeable blur, ask the patient to try and clear the print. If the patient can, continue to move the print closer to the eye until you reach the first sustainable blur and note this value.

9. Move the print slightly closer to the patient and then gradually move the target away and ask the patient to indicate when it just becomes clear. Note this point.

10. The amplitude of accommodation can be determined by taking the average of these two values. That is the point at which the target just gets blurred and the point at which it just becomes clear.

11. If the measured amplitude differs significantly from the normal values, repeat the test to ensure that the abnormal finding is not an artefact of the procedure.

Recording

Record the number of dioptres of accommodation for each eye and binocularly.

Interpretation

The figures in Table 4.1 are normal values of monocular spectacle accommodation. In the older age groups, as pupil size gets smaller and the actual amplitude reduces to zero (about 55 years), the measurements reflect the depth of focus rather than the amplitude of accommodation.

Table 4.1 Monocular expected accommodation levels as a function of age

Age (years)	Donders (D)	Duane (D)
10	14.00	11.00
15	12.00	10.25
20	10.00	9.50
25	8.50	8.50
30	7.00	7.50
35	5.50	6.50
40	4.50	5.50
45	3.50	3.50
50	2.50	
55	1.75	
60	1.00	1.25
65	0.50	
70	0.25	1.00
75	0.00	

Duane–Hoffstetter formula for probable amplitude of accommodation

$$25.0 - 0.40 \times \text{age Maximum amplitude}$$
$$18.5 - 0.30 \times \text{age Average amplitude}$$
$$15.0 - 0.25 \times \text{age Minimum amplitude}$$

If the measured amplitude is significantly lower than the normal values the patient may have an accommodative insufficiency (i.e. a functional loss that is not pathological or a paralysis/paresis of accommodation).

If the measured amplitude of accommodation is reduced due to the patient's age to a level below 5 D and the patient has difficulty reading, the patient has presbyopia.

Most common errors

1. Not making sure at the first reported blur that the patient has sufficient time to 'bring the print back into focus'.
2. Not stressing to the patient to report the first signs of blur, not when he or she can't read the text.
3. Moving the card too slowly and from too far away will tire the patient and can result in an artificially low score.
4. Moving the card too rapidly.

Further reading

London, R. (1991). Amplitude of accommodation. In *Clinical Procedures in Optometry* (J.B. Eskridge, J.F. Amos and J.D. Bartlett, eds) J.B. Lippincott, Philadelphia, Pennsylvania
Rosenfield, M. (1997). Accommodation. In *The Ocular Examination: Measurements and Findings* (K. Zadnik, ed.) W.B. Saunders, London, UK

Binocular status in the primary position (post-refraction)

Background

It is important to assess the patient's binocular status following refraction. The new refractive correction may change the binocular balance and could impair or improve oculomotor stability compared to the old prescription. This is particularly important for patients with an accommodative basis to their binocular vision problem as refractive adjustment often has a significant affect on binocular status.

Recommended test: Cover test. See Chapter 2.

Rationale

The cover test is the 'gold standard' test for the assessment of heterotropia and heterophoria. It is the only test which allows the clinician to distinguish between a heterophoria and a heterotropia. To assess the change in the heterophoria or heterotropia induced by the new Rx it is best to use the same procedure prior to and following refraction. Therefore, the recommended test in this case is the cover test as this is used before the refraction, either unaided or with the patient's own glasses. For assessment of heterotropia it is the most appropriate test for determination of the type and size of the deviation. Heterophoria size can be determined using a prism bar to neutralise the deviation. Assessment of heterophoria can also be performed using a number of tests which allow dissociation of the eyes.

Acceptable alternative procedures for heterophoria: Maddox rod and wing

Rationale

It is often difficult to perform the cover test when using reduced aperture trial case lenses or a phoropter, and in these situations the Maddox rod test (distance) and Maddox wing (near) provide simple and quick alternatives. Do not use these tests on patients who have a heterotropia. Dissociation tests allow the fusional vergence component of the overall response to be determined and are therefore only appropriate for use on patients with binocular vision. The Maddox rod and wing tests are probably the most commonly used tests by UK optometrists for measuring heterophoria. These are subjective tests which allow a numerical value to be quickly and simply given to the size of the deviation.

The Maddox rod is a distortion test as the subject views a spotlight with one eye and a distorted (red line) image with the other eye. As these images are different they are incapable of being fused by the visual system and hence the eyes adopt the fusion free position.

The Maddox wing achieves dissociation by presenting independent objects to the patient. As the images are dissimilar the incentive to fusion is abolished and the eyes adopt the fusion free position.

Distance heterophoria: Maddox rod

Procedure

Horizontal heterophoria

1. Ensure the patient is wearing his or her optimal distance refractive correction. Explain that you are going to determine how well their eye muscles work together with the new lenses.
2. Turn on the spotlight and place the Maddox rod in front of the right eye, making sure that the 'grooves' are absolutely horizontal. It is conventional to place the Maddox rod before the right eye.
3. Turn out the room lights.
4. Direct the patient to look at the distant spotlight, and ask the patient if the vertical red line is seen to the right, left or straight through the spotlight.
5. Some patients have difficulty seeing the red line initially. If they cannot see the red line, cover each eye in turn to demonstrate that one eye sees the spotlight and the other sees the red line. Once they are aware of the test format they are often able to see the red line and spotlight simultaneously. Placing a green filter before the eye viewing the spotlight also helps the patient perform the test. If difficulty is still experienced place the Maddox rod in front of the left eye and try again. If the spotlight and red line cannot be seen together then suppression may be present and follow-up tests should be performed.
6. With the Maddox rod in front of the right eye the following responses can occur (Figure 4.1):

   (a) If the line is seen to pass through the spotlight the patient has orthophoria.
   (b) If the line is to the left of the spotlight (crossed images) the patient has an exophoria. The size of the deviation is determined by placing base-in prisms before the left eye until the spotlight and red line are coincident.

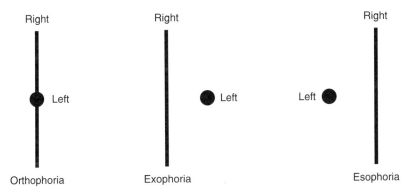

Figure 4.1 The relative positions of the red streak/line and white spot of light in orthophoria, exophoria and esophoria during Maddox rod measurement. The Maddox rod is placed before the right eye.

(c) If the line is to the right of the spotlight (uncrossed images) the patient has an esophoria. The size of the deviation is determined by placing base-out prisms before the left eye until the spotlight and red line are coincident.

7. As a screening technique, place a $2^\triangle$ prism with appropriate base direction in front of one eye. If the line now moves to the opposite side, the imbalance is within acceptable limits.

Vertical heterophoria
1. Rotate the Maddox rod do that the 'grooves' are absolutely vertical.
2. Ask the patient if the red line is seen above, below or straight through the spot.
3. With the Maddox rod in front of the right eye the following responses can occur (Figure 4.2):

   (a) If the line is seen to pass through the spotlight, the patient has orthophoria.
   (b) If the line is above the spotlight the patient has a right hypophoria. It is possible to specify vertical heterophorias with respect to the right or left eye. Thus, a right hypophoria can also be called a left hyperphoria. The size of the deviation is determined by placing base-down prisms before the left eye until the spotlight and red line are coincident.
   (c) If the line is to below the spotlight the patient has a right hyperphoria. This could also be called a left hypophoria. The size of the deviation is determined by placing base-up prisms before the left eye until the spotlight and red line are coincident.

4. It is also possible to record vertical heterophoria with respect to the higher eye. For example a $2^\triangle$ right hyperphoria can be specified as $2^\triangle$ R/L or a $3^\triangle$ right hypophoria can be specified as $3^\triangle$ L/R.

Most common errors

1. Allowing the patient to tip his or her head, either to the left or right, up or down.
2. Assessing muscle balance in a patient with no binocular function.

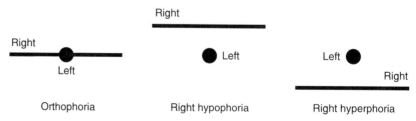

Figure 4.2 The relative positions of the red streak/line and white spot of light in orthophoria, right hypophoria and right hyperphoria during Maddox rod measurement. The Maddox rod is placed before the right eye.

3. Misinterpreting prism induced imbalance due to poorly centred lenses as a deviation.

Near heterophoria: Maddox wing

Procedure

1. Ensure the patient is wearing their optimal near refractive correction. If the patient is presbyopic, set the trial frame to the near PD.
2. Turn on the room lights and position an anglepoise lamp to provide additional illumination on the Maddox wing.
3. Direct the patient to look through the horizontal slits to view the chart which comprises horizontal and vertical scales and horizontal and vertical arrows. The right eye sees only the arrows whilst the left eye sees only the scales. The arrows are positioned at zero on the scales, but through dissociation any departure from orthophoria will be indicated by an apparent movement of the arrow along the scale.
4. Some patients have difficulty seeing the arrows and the scales simultaneously and require help to position the instrument correctly. If necessary, demonstrate that one eye views the arrows and the other eye views the scales. If the arrows and scales cannot be seen together then suppression may be present and follow-up tests should be performed.
5. Horizontal and vertical heterophorias can be measured with the Maddox wing.

   (a) To measure a *horizontal* heterophoria ask the patient: "Which white number does the white arrow point to?" The number on the scale indicates the magnitude of the deviation and the direction.

   (b) To measure a *vertical* heterophoria ask the patient: "Which red number does the red arrow point to?" The number on the scale indicates the magnitude of the deviation and the direction.

Most common errors

1. Allowing the patient to adopt an abnormal head position.
2. Assessing muscle balance in a patient with no binocular function.
3. Misinterpreting prism induced imbalance due to poorly centred lenses as a deviation.

Test limitations

1. The scale figures are too large to ensure accurate accommodation, which may lead to an overestimate of the exo deviation or underestimate of the eso deviation.
2. The septa do not allow the edge of the instrument to be fully dissociated, which may allow peripheral fusion to occur.

3. The tangent scale is designed for a standard PD.

Recording

1. The recording should be in prism dioptres. It should reflect the amount of prism and the direction the deviation, e.g. $3^{\triangle}$ SOP, $\cdot 5^{\triangle}$ XOP, $1^{\triangle}$ $\frac{R}{L}$, $\frac{1}{2}^{\triangle}$ $\frac{L}{R}$. If the screening technique was used, record < 2 XOP or $< \frac{1}{2}^{\triangle}$ $\frac{R}{L}$.
2. Note if any suppression took place during the test.

Interpretation

Each test of binocular status places the visual system under slightly different conditions, which makes absolute comparisons between tests difficult. The Maddox rod and Maddox wing are useful tests for measuring small to medium size heterophorias which can be performed under repeatable conditions. Most people with what we would consider as normal binocular vision have some slight degree of heterophoria. Approximately 1 to 2 prism dioptres of esophoria, or 1 to 4 prism dioptres of exophoria at distance, should be considered within the limits of normality. At near, 3 to 6 prism dioptres of exophoria is considered normal (physiological exophoria) and this can increase with age. With vertical phorias only about $\frac{1}{2}$ prism dioptre would be considered normal.

Further reading

Pickwell, L.D. (1989). *Binocular Vision Anomalies*, 2nd edn. Butterworths, London, UK

Stidwell, D. (1990). *Orthoptic Assessment and Management*. Blackwell Scientific Publications, Oxford, UK

Fixation disparity

Background

When viewing an object binocularly both visual axes are directed at the object of regard so that an image falls on the fovea of each eye. However, it is possible to fixate an object without the visual axes intersecting precisely on the object and still have binocular single vision providing the misalignment is within Panum's areas. A fixation disparity is present when one or both of the visual axes are not directed precisely on the fixation object.

If the visual axes are slightly divergent with respect to the fixation object there is an EXO disparity. If they are slightly convergent an ESO disparity is present. It is also possible to have vertical misalignment of the eyes which results in HYPER and HYPO disparities.

Fixation disparity is usually measured when the best refractive correction is in place. There are very few situations where measurement of fixation disparity unaided or with the patient's own Rx is useful. One such situation is when you find a small refractive error (Rx) or small change in Rx. If such a patient has non-specific symptoms, it can be difficult to decide whether to prescribe the small Rx/change in Rx. A finding of a fixation disparity unaided or with the patient's own Rx, and no disparity with the best refractive correction suggests that the new Rx/small change will benefit the patient and should be given.

Recommended test: Mallett unit

Procedure

Distance Mallett unit

1. Perform this test only on patients with binocular vision.
2. Seat the patient comfortably with the patient's head erect and eyes in the primary position of gaze. You should be directly in front of the patient so that you can view both eyes simultaneously, easily reach prisms and put the prisms in place.
3. Explain to the patient that this is a test which will help you determine whether his or her headaches (or whatever symptoms the patient has) could be due to a problem of the eye muscles not working together properly.
4. Turn on the Mallett unit, and put the OXO in a horizontal position with the red strips vertical. Keep the room lights on to illuminate the unit surroundings and provide paramacular and peripheral fusion stimuli.
5. Prior to placing the polaroid visa in front of the patient's eyes, ask the patient to: "Look at the X in the middle of the OXO; do you see two red strips, one above and one below the OXO? The two strips are in line with each other and in line with the middle of the X". This ensures that the patient is aware of what alignment looks like (Figure 4.3a), so that any misalignment is more obvious.
6. Place the polaroid visa in front of the patient's eyes and check that the top red strip is seen by the left eye, and the lower strip by the right eye.
7. Ask the patient: "Can you still see the two red strips?" If only one strip is seen, central suppression may be present, and no further measurement is possible. Most patients, however, should see both strips without difficulty.
8. Ask the patient: "Are the strips in line with the middle of the X?"
9. If both strips are seen to be aligned with X, no fixation disparity is present (Figure 4.3a).
10. If the lower red strip (RE) is to the left of the X and the upper strip (LE) is to the right, an exo disparity (uncompensated exophoria) is present in both eyes (Figure 4.3b).
11. If the lower strip (RE) remains below the X but the upper strip (LE) moves to the right, exo disparity is present in the left eye only (Figure 4.3c). When the disparity is unilateral, it is invariably the

Rationale

This is the most widely available test in the UK. The Mallett unit does not measure the size of the fixation disparity but helps determine the amount of prism required to reduce the fixation error to zero. The device has become popular in the UK as it is quick and easy to use and gives the prism or spherical lens power which can be used as the starting point for correction of binocular problems. The device has a central fixation lock (OXO) which allows the binocular status to be determined under natural viewing conditions. In the USA the Sheedy disparometer is more popular as it allows the size of the fixation disparity to be measured rather than the prism neutralisation point.

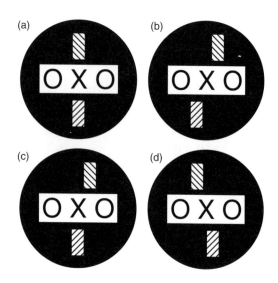

Figure 4.3 The positions of the red strips as seen by the patient with various types of fixation disparity. The lower strip is seen by the right eye and the top by the left eye. (a) No fixation disparity. (b) Lower strip (right eye) is seen to the left of the upper strip, indicating crossed disparity, i.e. exo disparity. (c) Exo disparity in the left eye only. (d) Eso disparity.

    non-dominant eye which demonstrates the deviation. Unilateral disparity is most common in vertical imbalance, whereas horizontal disparities are usually bilateral.

12. If an eso disparity is present, the lower strip (RE) will be to the right of the upper strip (LE) (Figure 4.3d).
13. The disparity is neutralised by the smallest prism or the weakest spherical lens which will reduce the disparity to zero. With a unilateral fixation disparity, add prism or spherical lenses to the eye demonstrating the slip. Between changes of prisms or lenses, instruct the patient to read a few Snellen letters from the distance chart.
14. Rotate the OXO into a vertical position with the red strips horizontal and repeat the assessment.

Mallett near unit

The Mallett near unit differs in the dimensions of the targets, the colour of the monocular strips (which are green as this is usually more sharply focused at *near* due to the slight lag of accommodation at near), and the presence of a paragraph of print surrounding the OXO which provides a peripheral fusion lock.

    The differences in the measurement are that the patient's normal reading spectacles or optimal near correction should be worn in the trial frame. The trial frame PD should be adjusted for near for presbyopes. A paragraph of small text must be read prior to any fixation disparity assessment to ensure accurate accommodation on the target.

Recording

If the two strips were not visible to the patient, always record which eye was suppressing and whether it was intermittent or constant. Use the suppression test on the Mallett unit to estimate the depth of the suppression. Record the lowest amount of prism and/or spherical lens required to align the strips.

Interpretation

The normal observer should be able to perceive both strips at all times. The strips are normally aligned without any prisms placed before the eyes. The size of the disparity (i.e. the amount of deviation of the monocular markers) is not *necessarily* proportional to the size of the phoria. A small heterophoria may give rise to a disparity, whilst a large phoria may be completely compensated (i.e. no disparity). The amount of prism required to reduce the disparity to zero is not *necessarily* proportional to the size of the disparity. Thus a fairly high amount of prism may be required to remove a small disparity.

The following general rules should be followed when treating a fixation disparity:

1. Only correct the fixation disparity if the patient has symptoms.
2. Prescribe prisms before the eye with the fixation disparity.
3. If the disparity is bilateral it is usual practice to split the prism between the two eyes.

There are 3 main ways of treating fixation disparity.

Exo-disparity

1. Prescribe the weakest base-in prism to neutralise the disparity. This is likely to be the best solution for adult patients.
2. Simulate accommodation and hence accommodate convergence by prescribing additional minus power. This approach only works in young patients.
3. Vision training can be employed to improve the positive fusional reserves to allow the patient to exert better control over the deviation.

Eso-disparity

1. Prescribe the weakest base-out prism to neutralise the disparity. This is likely to be the best solution for adult patients.
2. Accommodation can be relaxed for patients with a fixation disparity at near by prescribing a reading addition which will reduce the drive to accommodative convergence. This works well in younger patients but it is important that the add should never exceed the dioptric power of the working distance. The use of additional plus power is not a practical solution for distance disparities as the correction will blur distance vision.

3. Vision training can be employed to improve the negative fusional reserves to allow the patient to exert better control over the deviation. This option is usually best reserved for use in children.

Vertical disparity

Vertical disparity should only be treated with vertical prism. If horizontal and vertical disarity co-exist it is usual to correct the horizontal component first and reassess the vertical element. Any residual vertical component can then be corrected.

As vertical deviations frequently have an incomitant element it is essential that this diagnosis be considered during the examination.

Most common errors

1. Errors due to poorly fitting trial frame/phoropter or badly centred lenses.
2. Not starting with the lowest possible prism.
3. Taking too long to measure the associated phoria and allowing prism adaptation.
4. Not adjusting the instructions to the patient's age and capabilities.
5. Placing the prisms in the wrong direction.

Further reading

Mallett Unit Manual
Pickwell, L.D. (1989). *Binocular Vision Anomalies*, 2nd edn. Butterworths, London, UK
Stidwell, D. (1990). *Orthoptic Assessment and Management*. Blackwell Scientific Publications, Oxford, UK

Accommodative convergence/accommodation ratio (AC/A)

Background

Accommodation and convergence have a synkinetic relationship which ensures that clear, stable single binocular vision is present across a range of viewing distances. When accommodation (A) is exerted, the eyes are induced to converge, which is known as accommodative convergence (AC). The ratio of accommodative convergence to accommodation (AC/A) is a measure of how much accommodative convergence is induced (Δ) by one dioptre (D) of accommodation. This is a valuable measurement in the diagnosis and management of binocular vision anomalies where the AC/A may be abnormally high or low. The AC/A ratio normally remains almost constant throughout life until the onset of presbyopia. Measurements of AC/A after the age of 45 years are of little value.

Recommended test: Modified gradient

Procedure

1. Seat the patient comfortably. Ensure he or she is wearing an appropriate near correction (either the patient's own spectacles or the optimal near correction).
2. Give the patient the Maddox wing and ask the patient to hold it in a slightly depressed position, simulating a normal reading position. Sit slightly to one side of the patient, within easy reach of the trial case.
3. Keep the room lights on and direct the anglepoise over the patient's shoulder to evenly illuminate the Maddox wing.
4. Measure the horizontal heterophoria with the Maddox wing.
5. Insert +2.00 DS R and L and reassess the horizontal heterophoria.
6. Insert −2.00 DS R and L and reassess the horizontal heterophoria.
7. Use the following formula for each set of lenses to assess the AC/A and take an average:

$$AC/A = \frac{Heterophoria\ with\ minus\ lenses - Heterophoria\ with\ plus\ lenses}{Difference\ in\ power\ of\ lenses\ used}$$

Example: A patient has $14^\triangle$ esophoria with −2.00 D lenses R and L and $2^\triangle$ exophoria with +2.00 D lenses R and L. The AC/A ratio is calculated as below with esophoria being positive and exophoria being negative.

$$AC/A = \frac{14-(-2)}{2-(-2)}$$

$$= \frac{16}{4}$$

$$= 4^\triangle:1D$$

Rationale

The modified gradient test allows a quick and reliable measure of the AC/A ratio using basic clinical equipment. This procedure allows proximal components of the response to be controlled as the test is performed at a fixed distance. If a more precise measure of AC/A is required a full gradient test should be performed.

Interpretation

Normally the AC/A is $3–5^\triangle$/D. A low AC/A ratio may be indicative of a convergence insufficiency or convergence weakness problem. A high AC/A ratio may be indicative of a convergence excess problem or latent hyperopia. Knowledge of the AC/A ratio can be useful when determining lens power for the optical correction of convergence problems. As the amount of convergence induced by 1.00 D of accommodation is known, it is possible to calculate the initial lens power required to reduce the heterophoria to an acceptable level.

Most common errors

1. The result depends on heterophoria measures at only two points, which can lead to error. This problem can be overcome by performing the test using lenses between ±3.00 D in 1.00 D steps and plotting a

graph of lens power against induced heterophoria. The gradient of this line will give the AC/A ratio in $\triangle$/D.
2. Assuming that the test cannot be done when suppression is present.
3. Not adjusting the instructions to the patient's age and capabilities.
4. Not stimulating maximum accommodation effort.
5. Attempting the procedure on a presbyope.

Acceptable alternative technique: Heterophoria method

This test can be used routinely in practice to give a first estimate of the AC/A ratio as the information required is readily available following distance and near cover test or Maddox rod and wing testing. It does not allow proximal components of the accommodation and convergence responses to be controlled, which may lead to errors.

Procedure

1. Calculate the AC/A ratio as follows:

$$AC/A = PD + \frac{(n-d)}{D}$$

where PD = interpupillary distance in cm; n = near phoria; d = distance phoria; D = accommodation. Exophorias are negative and esophorias are positive. For example, PD = 6 and D = 2.5 (accommodation required from distance to 40 cm), distance phoria is ortho and near phoria is 5 exo, AC/A = 6 + (−5/2.5) = 4.

Advantages

The information is usually available during a routine eye examination and does not require any additional tests to be performed. A simple calculation can be performed using this information.

Disadvantages

1. Only two measures of heterophoria are used to calculate the AC/A.
2. Proximal accommodation is not controlled and influences the results. Using the gradient method the proximal component can be assumed to be constant as the test is performed at a fixed distance.

Further reading

Pickwell, L.D. (1989). *Binocular Vision Anomalies*, 2nd edn. Butterworths, London, UK
Stidwell, D. (1990). *Orthoptic Assessment and Management*. Blackwell Scientific Publications, Oxford, UK

Stereoacuity

Background

The fundamental characteristic of the type of binocular vision which has evolved in humans is stereoscopic vision. There are three anatomical and physiological requirements for stereoscopic vision: a large binocular overlap of the visual fields, partial decussation of the afferent visual fibres, and co-ordinated conjugate eye movements. Stereoscopic vision is absent in patients with strabismus and is either poor or absent in patients with amblyopia. Any obstacle to normal visual development early in life will be reflected in the level of stereoacuity attained.

Stereopsis is a useful method for evaluating the level of binocular vision present in children. Many tests are available which have different virtues. It is important to know the limitations of the test and the normal scores attainable for each age group. When conducting a test of stereopsis, ensure the patient wears the appropriate refractive correction.

Recommended test: TNO stereo

Procedure

1. Seat the patient comfortably. Ask the patient to wear the red–green diplopia goggles over the habitual correction. For the bifocal wearer, position the test properly for near-point viewing.
2. Instruct the patient to hold the book 40 cm from his or her face.
3. Keep the room lights on, and direct the anglepoise over the patient's shoulder to illuminate the booklet.
4. For a general screening test, the first four plates are used where the disparity is large and ungraded. Determine if the following can be seen by the patient:

   (a) Plate I. Ask the patient: "How many butterflies can you find on this page? Can you point to them?" There are two butterflies; one is seen monocularly and the other is seen only if stereopsis is present.

   (b) Plate II. Ask the patient: "How many circles? Which is the biggest?" There are four discs, of which two are seen with stereopsis.

   (c) Plate III. Ask the patient: "Can you find a cross/square/triangle/circle/diamond? Can you point to it?" Four 'hidden' shapes (circle, square, triangle, diamond) are arranged around a centrally easily visible cross. This plate is very useful with children as they like to find and name shapes.

   (d) Plate IV. Ask the patient: "How many circles can you see on this page? Can you point to them?" This is a suppression test. There are three discs; one seen with the right eye, one seen by the left eye, and one seen binocularly.

Rationale

An important requirement for stereoacuity tests is the removal of all monocular clues. If this requirement is fulfilled, judgements of depth will be made purely on the basis of the disparity between the two images. Each test plate of the TNO stereo test consists of a stereogram in which the images presented to each eye have been superimposed and printed in complementary colours. The stereograms are viewed through a pair of red and green filters. The stereograms are based on the random dot principle. Pairs of stereo-patterns composed of randomly arranged dots or squares are used, which viewed individually have no apparent depth. The obvious advantage of this type of test is that monocular clues are eliminated. The patient is required to describe the shape of the raised figure and, since this shape is only seen if stereopsis is present, there is no possibility of 'cheating'. This test can be performed well by children from the age of 3 years.

5. If plates I–IV are completed correctly, proceed to plates V to VII, which represent graded stereoacuities from 480 to 15 seconds of arc. Ask the patient: "In each of these squares there is a cake hidden with a piece missing. Can you find the cake and point to the piece that is missing?" For each test level, two discs with a sector missing are presented in different orientations.
6. If the patient is hesitant about an answer, allow plenty of time to view the test plate. If only one of the two tests for each acuity level is stated correctly, allow the patient a second attempt at the incorrect one, but if called incorrectly again, or if the patient cannot see a shape, record the stereoacuity as the previous correctly identified level.
7. Close the back and store in a light-free, dry environment.

Recording

1. If the stereo shapes are identified in plates I–III but not V–VII, record 'Gross stereopsis'.
2. If plate IV is identified incorrectly, record which is the suppressing eye.
3. For plates V–VII, record the stereoacuity as 'at least' the highest level where both responses were correct, e.g. 'Stereoacuity ≤ 15'.

Interpretation

If the stereo threshold is recorded as $\leq 40''$, one can assume that any ocular misalignments cannot be larger than Panum's fusional area. It is clinically acceptable for 60 sec of arc to be considered within normal limits. When the stereoacuity falls below 60 sec of arc, accurate bifoveal fixation cannot be assumed. However, in itself reduced stereoacuity does not specify a particular binocular disorder or its magnitude. Factors that could cause reduced stereoacuity are a small ocular misalignment, a small suppression scotoma, small amounts of blur (binocular, monocular) and/or aniseikonia.

Most common errors

1. Allowing the patient to change the working distance without altering the results accordingly.
2. Measuring stereopsis before the refraction with the patient's own spectacles, which may not be optimal.
3. Instructing the patient in such a manner that leads the patient to the answers.
4. Not allowing sufficient time for the patient to perceive the stereo figure.
5. Excessive glare on the page.
6. Not adjusting the instructions to the patient's age and capabilities.

Acceptable alternative procedures

Lang stereotest II (Random dot)

This test was designed to simplify stereopsis screening in children. It is based on two principles: random dots and cylindrical gratings. The test is a single card which can be held easily by the clinician or the patient. It has only three levels of stereopsis, which allow only gross stereopsis to be detected. With the test presented at 40 cm the patient has to locate the arc of the moon (200 sec), a star (200 sec), a car (400 sec) and an elephant (600 sec). The star can also be seen monocularly to help attract the attention of young children. Pre-verbal children respond by reaching for the images, an action which indicates that some stereopsis is present. This is a useful test to have available as it is easy to use, provides valuable information and is relatively inexpensive.

Advantages
1. No goggles required.
2. Appropriate for young children and infants (age 6 months or older). For very young children, eye movements should be observed as they can be used to indicate if the child is fixing a pattern in the same way as preferential looking is used to determine acuity level.

Disadvantages
1. Gross stereopsis only measurable.
2. Monocular cues available if the card is titled.

Frisby stereo test

The test uses sheets of perspex on to which are printed a random pattern of shapes. A circle within the pattern is printed on one face and the remainder of the pattern on the other face. The patient has to select the pattern which contains the circle in depth. The sheets of perspex are 1 mm, 3 mm and 6 mm thick and are presented at a range of fixation distances to achieve the necessary disparity. The test is usually used at 40 cm to start with, which allows a best stereoacuity of 85" to be measured. In theory, any disparity can be introduced by changing the fixation distance.

Advantages
1. Uses real depth rather than simulated depth.
2. Goggles not required (better for young children).
3. Infinite variation of stereo levels can be tested.
4. Durable test.

Disadvantages
1. Monocular cues with movement of the plate or patient's head. It is therefore important that the plate is displayed squarely and the patient's head kept still to minimise parallax effects.
2. Having to change working distance lenses for presbyopes.

Titmus fly test (Polaroid vectograph)

This is a popular clinical test which uses crossed Polaroid filters to present slightly different aspects of the same object to each eye. When the patterns are viewed through a Polaroid visor, the patterns are fused and seen in depth. The test has three sections. The circle patterns section provides the most sensitive assessment of stereopsis and should be used when possible.

1. The housefly, which manifests very large disparities, and should be seen in depth by most people. This part is particularly useful for young children, since they can be asked to touch the wing of the fly and their reaction noted.
2. Circle patterns. This section consists of a series of patterns each containing four circles. One of the circles in each group contains a graded disparity (crossed) so that when viewed binocularly, the circle is seen to 'float' in front of the others. The disparities of the circles range from 800 sec of arc to 40 sec. The patient is asked to indicate which one of the four circles stands out towards them.
3. Animals. There are three rows of animals, one animal in each row having a crossed disparity has to be identified by the patient. The disparities range from 400 to 100 sec. This section of the test is useful for young children.

Advantages
1. Most commonly available test.
2. The Titmus fly is a memorable test for all ages and popular (and useful) with children.

Disadvantages
1. The test contains potent monocular cues. Because all the disparities are crossed, the only possibility is that one circle will appear to lie in front of the others. The patient really only has to decide which circle is different. An intelligent subject could do this monocularly by observing which of the circles is slightly displaced.
2. Requires the use of a Polaroid visor.

Stereoacuity test on Mallett unit

Two vertical rows of geometric figures are viewed through a polarised visor and are fused by the patient. A $3^{\triangle}$ prism should be placed base-out in front of one eye to assist fusion of the two columns. The test measures acuities from 10 min of arc to 30 sec.

Advantages
1. Readily available in many UK optometric practices.
2. Can be performed at the same time as fixation disparity testing.

Disadvantages
1. Requires a Polaroid visor.
2. Difficult to instruct the patient, and shapes difficult to fuse.
3. Limited range of stereoacuities measured.

Fusional reserves

Background

Heterophorias are latent deviations which are corrected by the fusion reflex. A great deal of fusional effort may be required to correct a large heterophoria. It is important to know how much of the total fusional amplitude is required to correct the heterophoria and how much is kept in reserve. For reflex muscular activity, between $\frac{1}{3}$ and $\frac{2}{3}$ of the total amplitude may be used without placing the system under undue stress.

Positive and negative fusional reserves can be measured at distance and near by placing appropriate prisms before the eyes. Fusional reserve tests measure the amount of prism which can be introduced in front of the eyes before fusion breaks down and diplopia results. Placing base-out prism before the eyes causes the image of the stimulus to be deflected onto the temporal retina of each eye, which stimulates the eyes to converge. The amount of base-out prism required to produce diplopia is called the *positive fusional reserves*. Placing base-in prism before the eyes causes the image of the stimulus to be deflected onto the nasal retina of each eye, which stimulates the eyes to diverge. The amount of base-in prism required to produce diplopia is called the *negative fusional reserves*.

When changing the magnitude of prism placed before the eyes, three points should be noted:

1. The amount of prism required to *blur* the target (see below). This is called the *blur* point.
2. The amount of prism required to cause diplopia, which is called the *break* point.
3. The prism power should then be reduced until single vision is restored. This is known as the *recovery* point.

Blur point (positive and negative relative vergence)

When the eyes accommodate they also have a tendency to converge, which is known as accommodative convergence (AC). When the eyes converge they stimulate a certain amount of accommodation, which is known as convergence accommodation (CA). When measuring positive fusional reserves the target usually blurs before diplopia occurs. Because the eyes are forced to converge, accommodation is stimulated (CA) and cannot be maintained at the correct level of focus for the task. The amount of base-out prism to the blur point is known as positive relative accommodation. Measuring negative fusional reserves at near also induces blur prior to diplopia, as accommodation is forced to relax as the eyes diverge. The amount of base-in prism to the blur point is known as negative relative accommodation. It is not usual to obtain a blur point when measuring negative fusional reserves at distance, as accommodation is already at a minimum and cannot relax beyond this point.

Relative vergence represents the amount of convergence or divergence which can be induced to maintain fusion without changing accommodation. It is a measure of the flexibility of the linkage between accommodation and vergence.

Recommended test: Prism vergence in free space

Rationale

Free space methods most closely mimic natural viewing conditions and give a better indication of habitual visual function. This method is easy to perform and can be conducted easily in most clinics, as prism bars are often available. A variable prism stereoscope or a rotary prism are ideal methods of changing the amount of prism before the eyes in a smooth manner. However, these items are only available in most optometric practices in phoropters where they cannot be used to measure prism vergence in free space.

Procedure

Note: this description is for measurement at 6 m. The technique can be applied for near by adjusting the trial frame to the near interpupillary distance and positioning a fixation target at the appropriate position.

1. Seat the patient comfortably with his or her head erect and eyes in the primary position of gaze. The patient should wear his or her habitual correction; alternatively, the optimal correction can be placed in a trial frame. Keep the room lights on.
2. Position yourself in front of the patient so that you can view the patient's eyes easily, and enough to the side so that the patient's view of the target is not obstructed. Explain the procedure to the patient.
3. Isolate a single letter of a size equal to or slightly larger than the patient's visual acuity of the poorer eye. If a monocular visual acuity is less than 6/18, use a spotlight. At near a vertical line of letters is useful as a target.
4. Instruct the patient: "I would like you to look at the letter * at the other end of the room" (or "...the letter * on this stick" for near reserves).
5. Measure horizontal fusional reserves first. Position the prism bar so that horizontal prism will be introduced from a zero starting point over one eye.
6. Slowly increase the amount of prism placed before the eyes. Instruct the patient to report the first perceptible blur (with negative fusional reserves at distance there is not usually a blur point). As soon as the blur is reported, stop increasing the base-out prism and instruct the patient to attempt to clear the letters. If the letters can be cleared, continue to increase the prism slowly until the patient reports a blur that cannot be cleared. This is the sustained blur point. If the patient does not report a blur but instead reports diplopia first, then there is no blur point so record an 'X'.
7. Make a mental note of the prism amount before the patient's eye at the sustained blur point. Ask the patient to report when the letter

now doubles. Increase the amount of prism until the patient reports sustained double vision. This is the break point.

8. After making a mental note of the prism before the eye when the patient reports doubling, increase slightly the amount of prism to ensure complete separation of the doubled image. The patient's vergence eye movements should be noted objectively by the practitioner.
9. If the amount of prism that has been added seems unusually large, ask the patient if the letters have remained centred or if they have drifted off to the side. If they have drifted, this indicates that one eye has been suppressed. The direction of movement will indicate which eye has been suppressed. A versional (as opposed to vergence) eye movement will be seen objectively.
10. Slowly reduce the amount of prism until the patient reports that the two images have moved together into a single image. This is the recovery point. Make a mental note of the amount of prism in front of the patient's eye and remove the prism bar.

Recording

1. NFR: X/14/10
2. PFR: 12/18/10
3. BU/OS + VR: 3/1
4. BD/OS − VR: 3/1
5. If base-out prism has to be employed to acquire a measure of the negative fusional reserves (NFR) record the value as minus, i.e. X/−10/−14. This would indicate that 14 base-out was required to acquire single vision and that the base-out prism was reduced to 10 to measure the amount of NFR. Conversely, negative (minus) values are used if base-in prism has to be employed to acquire a measure of the positive fusional reserves (PFR). Similarly, negative values may be recorded with vertical vergences.
6. If the limits of the prism are met, record as > 40 (or the maximum prism value).

Interpretation

Table 4.2 shows the normal range of fusional reserves. A patient with an exophoria will use part of the positive fusional amplitude to correct the deviation. The measured positive fusional reserves therefore represent the amount of fusional vergence in reserve to maintain single vision. A patient with esophoria will use part of the negative fusional amplitude to correct the deviation. The measured negative fusional vergence represents the amount of remaining fusional vergence. A knowledge of the heterophoria size and the magnitude of the relevant fusional reserves can be useful in the assessment of a patient's binocular status. The proportion of the total fusional vergence used to correct the heterophoria can be determined. For example:

Table 4.2 Normal range of fusional reserves

	Distance (range Δ)	Near (range Δ)
Positive fusional reserves		
Blur	12–16	20–28
Break	18–22	26–34
Recovery	14–18	22–30
Negative fusional reserves		
Blur	Not applicable	6–10
Break	6–12	12–18
Recovery	4–8	8–14

Distance heterophoria 9^{Δ} exophoria

Positive fusional reserves 18^{Δ}

Total positive fusional amplitude $18^{\Delta} + 9^{\Delta} = 27^{\Delta}$

Therefore, one third of the total positive fusional vergence is used to correct the heterophoria which is within normal limits.

This approach has been formalised in Sheard's and Percival's rules which are used to compare the fusional reserves with the heterophoria and indicate whether the heterophoria is decompensated.

Vertical fusional reserves

To measure vertical fusional reserves it is necessary to place base-up prism before one eye and base-down prism before the other eye until fusion is broken. Break and recovery points should be recorded. A blur point is not reached when measuring vertical fusion. When base-down prism is placed before the right eye and base-up before the left eye (right eye moves up and left eye moves down), this provides a measure of right supravergence and left infravergence.

It should be noted that the magnitude of vertical fusional reserves is considerably less than horizontal.

Most common errors

1. Asking for a blur point with the vertical vergences or negative fusional vergence at distance.
2. Assuming that the test can be done when suppression is present, such as with a strabismic condition.
3. Not adjusting the instructions to the patient's age and capabilities.
4. Not providing appropriate stimulus to accommodation, either by an inappropriate correction or poor accommodative target.
5. Not ensuring that the patient is looking through the centre of the prism rather than through the strips separating the prisms.

Pickwell, L.D. (1989). *Binocular Vision Anomalies*, 2nd edn. Butterworths, London, UK
Stidwell, D. (1990). *Orthoptic Assessment and Management*. Blackwell Scientific Publications, Oxford, UK

Degree of incomitancy

Background

The pen torch motility test is useful in the initial diagnosis of incomitant strabismus but has limitations in allowing the paretic muscle to be identified reliably. To allow a specific diagnosis it is necessary to perform a more precise test which dissociates the eyes and allows a comparison of primary and secondary angles in all positions of gaze. The most popular or commonly used tests are the Hess screen and the Lees screen.

Recommended test: Hess screen

Procedure

1. Seat the patient upright with his or her head erect and eyes in the primary position, eyes level with the central point of the Hess screen, and accurately positioned 50 cm away from the screen. The test can be performed wearing a spectacle correction provided the lens size is large and no bifocals are worn. If the frame or lenses cause a restriction in the field of view then remove the refractive correction. Ask the patient to put on the 'wrap-around' red–green diplopia goggles. Give the patient the focused green pen torch.
2. Sit or stand behind the patient holding the board with mounted recording chart and remote control.
3. Dim the room lights to a level where the patient cannot see the markings on the Hess screen through the goggles but you can see them to record the results.
4. Determine which eye is viewing though the red filter (the fixing eye) and select the appropriate half of the recording chart.
5. Switch on one of the red lights. Instruct the patient: "Please keep your head absolutely still and in the straight ahead position. When you see a red light, try to cross it with your green light, and tell me when it is crossed".
6. Mark with a dot on the chart where the centre of the green slit is positioned when the patient tells you it has crossed the red light.
7. Repeat this for each of the inner nine red lights. There is no particular order of presentation. If necessary, use the outer scale to plot additional points.

Rationale

The Hess plot represents an accurate method of assessing the deviation of the visual axes in different positions of gaze. It is a wall mounted flat screen which fits conveniently into a consulting room. The Lees screen is more widely used in hospitals as the patient does not need to wear goggles and the viewing simulates free space. However, this test requires a relatively large amount of space and is expensive to purchase. These factors have restricted its use in optometric practice.

8. Repeat the procedure with the goggles reversed, taking care to record on the other half of the recording chart. By placing the red glass before the other eye fixation is changed. This allows the appropriate comparison of movements to be considered.

9. When the test has been completed join each of the dots of the inner box together with a straight line. If necessary, join the outer points together with a straight line.

Interpretation

Compare the plots obtained with the right and left eyes fixating. Plots of equal size and without distortion indicate that the deviation (which may be a heterophoria or heterotropia) is comitant, and those corresponding exactly with the pre-printed lines on the chart indicate that the patient is orthophoric. Plots which are of unequal size indicate that the deviation is incomitant, and the smallest plot indicates the affected eye. The point furthest from its origin indicates the affected muscle. Confirmation of the diagnosis is achieved by following the ocular sequelae of muscle paresis:

1. Greatest underaction of the affected muscle.
2. Overaction of the contralateral synergist.
3. Overaction (contracture) of the ipsilateral direct antagonist.
4. Secondary inhibition of the contralateral antagonist.

Most common errors

1. Not keeping the patient's head still.
2. Plotting the points on the wrong half of the chart.
3. Not wrapping the goggles properly around the patient's eyes, thus allowing the patient to look through the filters in extremes of gaze.

Acceptable alternative procedure: Prism cover test

Procedure

1. Perform a prism cover test at arm's length in the primary position and in each of the nine positions of gaze. An accommodative target should be used with the patient corrected for the appropriate distance.
2. Record the results in a 'noughts and crosses' diagram.

Advantage

Full dissociation of the eyes is achieved.

Disadvantages

1. Difficult to perform accurately.
2. Interpretation of results is more difficult than with the Hess screen plots.

Further reading

Pickwell, L.D. (1989). *Binocular Vision Anomalies*, 2nd edn. Butterworths, London, UK

Stidwell, D. (1990). *Orthoptic Assessment and Management*. Blackwell Scientific Publications, Oxford, UK

5
Ocular health assessment

Pupillary function

Background

Evaluation of pupillary function provides valuable information about the integrity and function of the iris, optic nerve, posterior visual pathways and the third and sympathetic nerves to the eye. Afferent pupillary defects are caused by lesions in the 'front end' of the pupillary light reflex pathway and most commonly lesions in the retina and optic nerve. The afferent pupillary pathways leave the visual pathways in the last third of the optic tracts to reach the pretectal nuclei. Afferent pupillary defects do not cause anisocoria (different pupil sizes), but may produce abnormal pupillary light reflexes. Efferent pupillary defects produce anisocoria and are caused by lesions to the motor neurone system which carries signals from the central nervous system to the iris.

> **Recommended tests: Direct measurement of pupil size in dim and bright illumination, direct and consensual pupil light reflexes and swinging flashlight test**

Procedure

1. Ask the patient to take off his or her glasses, and look at a letter on the Snellen chart which both eyes can see easily. If the worst monocular visual acuity is less than about 6/18, ask the patient to look at a spot of light on the distance chart.
2. Sit in front and to the side of the patient, so that you can easily observe the patient's pupils, but you are not obscuring his or her fixation of the Snellen chart.
3. Keep the room lights on and check the size, shape and location of both pupils. Compare the size of both pupils very carefully. Black semicircles on rulers (or on the Keeler specialist ophthalmoscope) are preferred over simple millimetre rulers.
4. Dim the room lights but keep the light levels high enough so that you can easily see the patient's pupils, and compare the size of the

Rationale

These tests are quick and simple and can be performed without the need for any additional equipment. Pupil size should be assessed in both bright and dim illumination to investigate any anisocoria. The swinging flashlight provides a sensitive assessment of any unilateral or asymmetric afferent defects. There is no condition in which the near reflex is defective or lost when the light reflex is normal. Therefore the near reflex need only be checked if the light reflex is abnormal.

patient's pupils again. A Burton lamp can be used with patients with very dark irides.

5. Direct and consensual light reflexes:

   (a) Ask the patient to remain fixating a letter or spotlight on the distance chart.
   (b) Shine a pen light or direct ophthalmoscope into the right pupil from the inferior temporal side from a distance of 5 to 10 cm. Observe the extent and speed of constriction of the right pupil (direct light reflex) and left pupil (consensual reflex). Check this several times as dramatic fatigue can occur in an abnormal eye which at first shows a normal response.
   (c) Remove the light and observe the direct and consensual dilation.
   (d) Repeat the observations while shining the light into the left pupil.

6. Swinging flashlight test (or Marcus–Gunn pupil):

   (a) Ask the patient to remain fixating a letter or spotlight on the distance chart.
   (b) Shine a pen light or direct ophthalmoscope into the right eye from below the patient's eyes from a distance of 5 to 10 cm. Pause for 2–3 sec and then quickly switch the light to shine into the left eye.
   (c) Repeatedly alternate between the two eyes, pausing for 2–3 sec on each eye, and look for any change in pupil size as the light is alternated.
   (d) An eye with a relative afferent pupillary defect will dilate as the eye is turned upon it, as the consensual dilation response due to the light moving off the other good eye overpowers the poor constriction response from the affected eye.

7. Near reflex. There is no condition in which the near reflex is defective or lost when the light reflex is normal. Therefore the near reflex need only be checked if the light reflex is abnormal.

   (a) Ask the patient to remain fixating a letter or spotlight on the distance chart.
   (b) Ask the patient to then look at a target such as the patient's own thumb about 15 cm from his or her eyes.
   (c) Observe the extent and speed of pupillary constriction as the patient changes fixation from distance to near.
   (d) Ask the patient to look back at the distance target and observe the dilation as this occurs.

Recording

Record the size and shape of the pupils, and particularly note any anisocoria. The acronym PERRL (Pupils Equal Round and Respond to Light) can be used or a 0 to 4+ grading system where:

0   indicates no pupil response
1+ indicates a very small, just visible response
2+ indicates a small, slow response
3+ indicates a moderate response
4+ indicates a brisk, large response typical of a healthy young patient.

If the light reflex is abnormal, the near reflex must be checked. Some disorders produce an absent light reflex with a normal near reflex (light–near dissociation).

Also record a positive or negative swinging flashlight test or Marcus–Gunn pupil. A negative result indicates that there is no problem. If a positive swinging flashlight test is found, record which side was defective.

Interpretation

Pupils are normally equal in size and vary from 2 to 4 mm in diameter in bright light to about 4 to 8 mm in dim light. The pupil gets smaller with age and shows physiological fluctuations in size or hippus. Physiological anisocoria is not uncommon (≥ 0.5 mm of anisocoria is seen in about 20% of normal patients). Physiological anisocoria is generally the same in dim and bright illumination, is usually small (< 1 mm), has been present for years (i.e. can be seen on old photographs) and shows normal pupil reflexes.

Pathological anisocoria is due to an abnormality in the efferent or motor pupil pathway. Anisocoria which is greater in dim illumination than in bright light could be due to Horner's syndrome, although some cases of physiological anisocoria can show this feature. In both cases the light reflexes are normal, but the dilation of the affected eye in dim illumination is much slower in Horner's syndrome. For definitive differential diagnosis, pharmacological tests are necessary. Anisocoria which is greatest in bright light will generally show an abnormal direct and consensual light reflex. This indicates a problem in the motor leg of the light reflex pathway, such as in the third nerve, ciliary ganglion or iris, or could be drug induced.

An abnormal direct light response in a pupil capable of a normal consensual response indicates an afferent (visual pathway) defect. There is generally no anisocoria. The swinging flashlight provides a more sensitive assessment of any unilateral or asymmetric afferent defects. It compares each eye's direct response (reflecting the normality of its visual pathway) with its consensual response (reflecting the normality of the other eye's visual pathway). Symmetrical afferent defects do not show a positive Marcus–Gunn pupil.

Most common errors

1. Forgetting to check pupil reflexes prior to instilling a mydriatic or cycloplegic.
2. Using too low a light level to observe the contralateral eye, especially with a darkly pigmented eye.

3. Blocking the patient's view of the Snellen chart and stimulating accommodation and subsequent pupil constriction.
4. Using too slow a swing in the swinging flashlight test.

Further reading

Friedman, N.E. (1997). The pupil. In The *Ocular Examination: Measurements and Findings* (K. Zadnik, ed.) W.B. Saunders, London, UK

London, R. and Eskridge, J.R. (1991). Pupil evaluation. In *Clinical Procedures in Optometry* (J.B. Eskridge, J.F. Amos, J.D. Bartlett, eds) J.B. Lippincott, Philadelphia, Pennsylvania

Anterior segment examination

Background

The purpose of anterior segment examination is to detect abnormalities or anomalies of the eyelids, conjunctiva, tear layer, cornea, anterior chamber, iris, crystalline lens and anterior vitreous. This procedure should be performed as a routine test during all primary care assessments, during all contact lens assessments and during problem specific assessments involving the anterior segment or adnexa. However, note that the PQE 'routine' examination requires an assessment of the anterior segment using a direct ophthalmoscope or loupe examination.

Recommended test: Slit lamp biomicroscopy examination

Rationale

Slit lamp biomicroscopy examination provides variable magnification under controlled illumination conditions. It is preferred over direct ophthalmoscopy, pen light technique or Burton lamp assessment because it provides greater magnification and resolution and greater control of illumination. Biomicroscopes can be attached to an arm of the examination stand or can be free standing on an examination table. For infants and patients using a wheelchair, a hand-held biomicroscope is the best option.

Procedure

Learn to adjust the biomicroscope before the examination begins. The positions of the controls differ for different models but all models have similar features. It should be possible to change the width of the beam, change the height of the beam, rotate the beam, change the angle between the light source and the viewing system, add filters over the light source, change the magnification (this may involve changing the eyepieces to a stronger power), change the intensity of the illumination, adjust the height of the microscope, focus the microscope with the joystick and, with most instruments, break the linkage between the illumination and viewing systems.

If one is available, place the focusing rod in the appropriate holder, with the flat surface towards you. Adjust the distance between the eyepieces to match your PD, and focus each eyepiece individually. If you are emmetropic or corrected with contact lenses this should be at the zero marking on the eyepiece. If you are not emmetropic, you may find the range of focus of the biomicroscope to be better if the eyepieces are adjusted to match your spherical refractive error. Normally, biomicroscope examination is performed uncorrected, as the field of view is greater the closer your eyes are to the eyepieces. If you have a high cylinder in your spectacle correction, you may need to wear your glasses to obtain adequate resolution.

1. Seat the patient comfortably on a stable chair without rollers, and ask the patient to remove any spectacles. You should be comfortably seated on the other side of the instrument. Explain the procedure in lay terms to your patient.
2. Adjust the height of the biomicroscope table/arm so that the patient may lean forward comfortably and place his or her chin in the rest. Adjust the chin rest so that the patient's eyes are at an appropriate height to provide a large enough vertical range to allow adequate examination of the adnexa. Many biomicroscopes have an eye alignment marker on the supporting beam of the head rest that can be used to judge this height. It should be level with the patient's outer canthus.
3. Dim the room lights and ask the patient to look at your ear or the instrument's fixation device. These are appropriate targets to get the patient's eyes in the primary position of gaze.
4. Use one hand to control the joystick (focusing) and the other to control the magnification and illumination and to manipulate the patient's lids.

There are several different types of illumination that can be used alternately or in combination to examine the anterior segment and adnexa. Using these methods of illumination the external eye and adnexa can be examined thoroughly.

5. Use *diffuse illumination* by adjusting the illumination to a wide beam and placing a diffusing filter in front of it. Use low magnification and make an overall assessment of the anterior segment. Ask the patient to close the lids and make a 'sweep' of the superior lid, paying special attention to the lashes and lid margins.
6. Ask the patient to open his or her eyes and examine the cornea and conjunctiva with a *parallelepiped* by setting the illumination system at approximately 45° from the microscope position and using a beam width of approximately 2 mm. An illuminated block of corneal tissue in the shape of a parallelogram should be visible. Use low to moderate magnification, as magnification that is too high will result in missing obvious, moderately sized abnormalities. Examine the temporal cornea first with the illumination coming from the temporal side. Move the beam laterally across the cornea until the centre of the cornea is reached. Then sweep the illumination system across to the nasal side, taking care not to bump the patient's nose, and examine the nasal cornea. You should look at both the area illuminated (direct illumination) and the area just outside the area of illumination (indirect illumination). If required, you can increase the width of the section of stroma seen by increasing the angle between the microscope and illumination system. You can also obtain greater detail by increasing the magnification.

Ask the patient to look in right and left gaze to expose the conjunctiva and the caruncle. Next, ask the patient to look upwards while the lower lid is gently pulled downward to expose the lower fornix. Then ask the patient to look downwards and gently pull the upper lid up, thereby exposing the superior cornea for examination. Finally, inspect the iris and crystalline lens.

7. If an abnormality/anomaly is detected use one or more of the following illumination techniques as appropriate (with experience, many or all techniques are used in fast succession). Vary the magnification to examine the anomaly more carefully, noting its exact size, shape, appearance, depth and location.

   (a) *Sclerotic scatter* (Figure 5.1) allows the observation of central corneal clouding, especially due to polymethyl methacrylate (PMMA) contact lens wear. Scars and foreign bodies on the cornea that cause light to scatter are also easily observable.

   Set the illumination system at 45° or greater from the observation system and direct the light onto the limbus. Break the linkage between the illumination and observation systems ("uncoupling"). With the light directed onto the limbus, you can now look through the eyepieces using low magnification and focus on the cornea. The light creates total internal reflection in the cornea and a glowing ring of light is created around the limbus. Anything blocking the transparency of the cornea

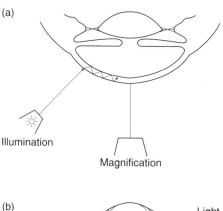

Illumination

Magnification

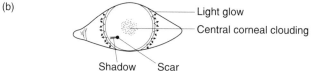

Light glow

Central corneal clouding

Shadow   Scar

Figure 5.1 (a) The technique of sclerotic scatter used with a biomicroscope. (b) The observation of central corneal clouding and a corneal scar using this technique. (Reprinted with permission from Hrynchak, P. (1996). *Procedures in Clinical Optometry*. University of Waterloo Press, Waterloo, Canada).

can be observed through the microscope against the dark backdrop of the pupil. You may find the observation easier by viewing the cornea without looking through the biomicroscope.

(b) *Direct illumination.* In this method the illumination beam and viewing system are sharply focused on the same area. There are three basic types of direct focal illumination:

  (i) Parallelepiped: used in the routine examination (see above).

  (ii) Optical section: used to look at opacities in the stroma and epithelium and to judge their depth, e.g. scars, infiltrates, dystrophies, corneal nerves, blood vessels, foreign bodies, etc. Set the illumination system at approximately $45°$ from the microscope using low to moderate magnification. Narrow the beam to the narrowest possible width and sharply focus on the cornea using the joystick. A section or 'slice' of the cornea should now be visible. The width of the section of stroma being seen can be increased by increasing the angle between the microscope and illumination system. Once the object of interest is identified, greater detail can be obtained by increasing the magnification.

  (iii) Conical beam: used to look for flare (i.e. protein) or floating cells in the anterior chamber by using more magnification and a longer beam. Turn off all the room lights and start to dark adapt. Set the illumination system at approximately $45°$ from the microscope using low to moderate magnification. Narrow the height and width of the beam to obtain a conical beam. Move the beam to the centre of the pupil and focus in the anterior chamber midway between the anterior surface of the crystalline lens and the posterior surface of the cornea. Rock the illumination system gently from side to side and look for flare/cells, etc. This technique is also discussed in the superficial conjunctional and corneal foreign body section.

(c) *Indirect illumination* (Figure 5.2): used to view areas that become bleached with excessive light using direct illumination, such as fine blood vessels at the limbus and microcysts. Also used to look for iris pathology. Use a parallelepiped and set the illumination system at a wide angle from the microscope and focus on an area adjacent to the area of observation. This can be done by rotating the prism or reflecting mirror. More simply, you can merely direct your gaze just outside the area that is illuminated. The magnification may be varied depending on the structure being viewed.

(d) *Retro-illumination* (Figure 5.3): used in the examination of corneal vessels, epithelial oedema, and small scars on the cornea as well as vacuoles and cataracts in the crystalline lens. It can also be used to detect the loss of pigment in the iris which occurs in albinism or pigmentary dispersion glaucoma (i.e. iris

(a)

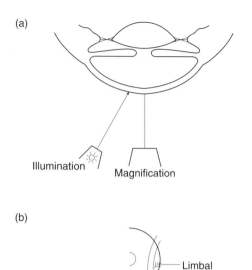

(b)

Figure 5.2 (a) The technique of indirect illumination used with a biomicroscope. (b) Limbal blood vessels (neovascularisation) seen using this technique. (Reprinted with permission from Hrynchak, P. (1996). *Procedures in Clinical Optometry*. University of Waterloo Press, Waterloo, Canada.)

(a)

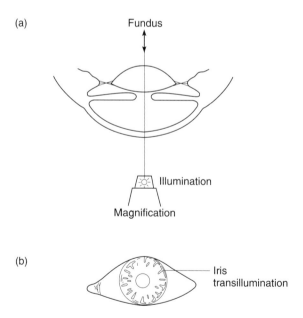

(b)

Figure 5.3 (a) The technique of retro-illumination used with a biomicroscope. (b) The observation of iris transillumination in an albino using retro-illumination from the fundus. (Reprinted with permission from Hrynchak, P. (1996). *Procedures in Clinical Optometry*. University of Waterloo Press, Waterloo, Canada.)

transillumination). Opaque features appear dark against a light background.

Set the illumination system at approximately 60° from the microscope, and use a parallelepiped with low magnification. Look through the eyepieces and use the joystick to focus on the structure to be examined against the light reflected from either the iris, the lens or the retina. If indirect retroillumination is desired, the object of interest is not viewed in the direct pathway of the reflected light, but rather against a dark non-illuminated background by breaking the linkage between the magnification and illumination systems, or by shifting the examiner's gaze to this area. The magnification can be varied as necessary.

(e) *Specular reflection* (Figure 5.4): used to examine the endothelium for polymegathism and pleomorphism, the precorneal tear film and variations in contour of the epithelium. Set the illumination system at approximately 45° to 60° from the microscope, using a moderately wide parallelepiped. Look through the eyepieces and focus the parallelepiped on the cornea. Change the angle of illumination until a bright reflection is seen from the precorneal tear film. This occurs when the angle of incidence equals the angle of reflection from the cornea. This can also be obtained by moving the illumination/microscope system laterally until the angle of incidence equals the angle of reflection. The precorneal

(a)

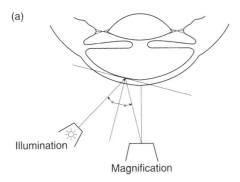

Illumination

Magnification

(b)

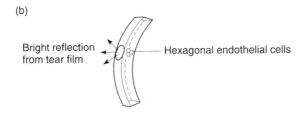

Bright reflection from tear film

Hexagonal endothelial cells

Figure 5.4 (a) The technique of specular reflection used with a biomicroscope. (b) The observation of the endothelial mosaic with specular reflection and high magnification. (Reprinted with permission from Hrynchak, P. (1996). *Procedures in Clinical Optometry*. University of Waterloo Press, Waterloo, Canada.)

tear film and epithelium can then be examined. To examine the endothelium set the magnification to 30–40× with a fairly wide parallelepiped. Focus to the back of the parallelepiped and a fairly small area of hexagonal cells should become apparent. If the bright reflection from the tear film interferes with the observation, try changing the width of the beam or increasing the angle of observation.

Recording

Record the size, shape, appearance and location of any abnormalities/anomalies using a diagram and a written description. Photo-documentation of significant abnormalities should be used when available. If no abnormalities are detected, this should be recorded.

Grading of opacification of the crystalline lens. The crystalline lens should be graded on a scale of 0 to 4^+ with 0 being absence of opacity and 4^+ being the most severe form of opacity. For more precise grading, a cataract grading system such as the LOCS III system should be used.

Grading of positive biomicroscope findings. Other positive biomicroscope findings should be graded on a scale of 0 to 4^+ with 0 being absence of a response, 1^+ trace response, 2^+ being mild response, 3^+ being moderate response and 4^+ being severe response. Observations such as stippling, corneal oedema, flare, tarsal plate abnormalities, injection and vascularisation should all be graded.

Interpretation

The examiner must have an adequate understanding of the normal anatomy and physiology of the cornea and anterior segment and normal change with healthy ageing to judge the health of the examined tissues.

Most common errors

1. Not focusing the eyepieces to compensate for the examiner's refractive error.
2. Not reducing the room illumination for the procedure.
3. Not examining the superior cornea by having the patient look down and raising the upper lid.
4. Exaggerating the appearance of the pathology in the recording.

Supplementary procedures

Lid eversion

Lid eversion is used to examine the superior palpebral conjunctiva. Ask the patient to look down and grasp the superior lashes. Use a cotton swab (or the index finger of the other hand) to press gently on the superior margin of the tarsal plate, and at the same time pull the lashes upwards. This technique will evert the lid to permit viewing the palpebral conjunctiva. To re-evert the lid hold the lashes and ask the patient to look up and gently pull the lashes away from the eye.

Fluorescein staining

Fluorescein staining is used to assess the integrity of the corneal epithelium as it accumulates in epithelial defects. See Diagnostic drugs section below for the full procedure. Wet the tip of a fluorescein strip with sterile saline solution. Be careful not to contaminate the saline by touching the strip to the tip of the bottle. Touch the strip to the inferior or superior bulbar conjunctiva while the patient looks away and the examiner holds the lid away from the eye. Ask the patient to blink several times. Observe the cornea with cobalt blue light and medium magnification. A Kodak Wratten number 12 yellow gelatin filter held in front of the biomicroscope viewing system will facilitate the view by filtering out the reflected blue light. Observations should be made within 10 min of instillation of the dye or intercellular diffusion surrounding a lesion may mask its exact nature. Soft contact lens wearers can replace their lenses after a biomicroscopic investigation using fluorescein as long as the dye is irrigated out of the eye using saline prior to lens reinsertion.

Rose Bengal staining

Rose Bengal staining is used to help diagnose a dry eye as it stains dead and devitalised cells bluish red or red. See Diagnostic drugs section below for the full procedure. Ask the patient to blink several times. Observe with white light and medium magnification within 5 min of instillation of the dye.

Tear break-up time

Tear break-up time (BUT) is used to assess the stability of the tear film and is a useful test for dry eye. With the patient at the biomicroscope, instil fluorescein into the eyes and ask the patient to blink several times, then to hold their eyes open without blinking. Scan the cornea with a parallelepiped and low magnification and time how long it takes before dark spots or streaks in the even green tear film appear. The use of the Kodak Wratten yellow filter number 12 is helpful for this evaluation. The normal break-up time is between 15 and 45 sec and a break-up time of less than 10 sec is indicative of an unstable tear film. If the tear film breaks up immediately and consistently in the same location there may be an epithelial basement membrane defect in that spot. The BUT should be repeated, not considering this defect, to get an indication of tear film stability. Do not use an anaesthetic prior to BUT measurement, as they can cause a spuriously fast BUT.

Further reading

Bartlett, J.D. (1991). Slit lamp. In *Clinical Procedures in Optometry* (J.B. Eskridge, J.F. Amosand and J.D. Bartlett, eds) J.B. Lippincott, Philadelphia, Pennsylvania

Catania, L.J. (1995). *Primary Care of the Anterior Segment.* Appleton and Lange Norwalk, Connecticut

Yolton, D.P. (1991). Topical ophthalmic dyes. In *Clinical Procedures in Optometry* (J.B. Eskridge, J.F. Amos and J.D. Bartlett, eds) J.B. Lippincott, Philadelphia, Pennsylvania

Direct fundus examination

Background

The invention of the ophthalmoscope revolutionised ocular health examination by allowing examination of the fundus and replacing the diagnosis of 'amaurosis' (an outwardly healthy eye with poor vision) with a multitude of others for which an aetiology and treatment could be sought. Direct fundus examination provides information on the clarity of the ocular media and integrity of the posterior pole, retinal vasculature and optic nerve head. Abnormalities or anomalies such as naevi, macular haemorrhages, optic nerve cupping, etc. may be assessed with this technique.

Recommended test: Direct ophthalmoscopy

Rationale

Direct ophthalmoscopy is used mainly when the pupil is not dilated to obtain a view of the fundus. It has the advantage of being a simple technique to perform, providing an erect view of the fundus with moderate magnification, can be performed on a non-dilated pupil and can be easily performed with the patient sitting upright. The equipment required is also less costly than for alternative techniques. The disadvantages are that it does not allow a stereoscopic view of the fundus, the extent of the fundus that is visible is limited, and the field of view is also limited. There is a variation in magnification with refractive error such that increasing amounts of myopia

Procedure

Familiarise yourself with the controls of the direct ophthalmoscope. Learn how to vary the intensity of the light beam, its size, shape and colour. Some instruments also have settings that will project a target with the light beam. Determine how to focus the outcoming light from the patient's fundus with the wheel of lenses. For most ophthalmoscopes, the red numbers indicate minus lenses and the black numbers indicate plus lenses. Some instruments have a second wheel of lenses or setting for additional lenses that, when used in combination with the first wheel of lenses, allow for higher total dioptric power in the instrument.

1. Seat the patient comfortably in the examination chair with his or her head held upright. The chair should be raised to such a position that you can comfortably look into the patient's eye (from the patient's temporal side) by bending over only slightly. If you or the patient is ill a face mask may be advisable. Inform the patient that you are going to examine the health of their eyes.

2. Set the ophthalmoscope to a mid-sized, white beam of moderate intensity, with about a $+8.00\,D$ lens (plus your refractive error, i.e. a $-6.00\,D$ myope should start with a $+2.00$ lens) in the lens wheel.

3. Ask the patient to remove his or her spectacles and remove your own. If you have an unusually large astigmatic or myopic correction it may be necessary to wear spectacles or contact lenses while using the direct ophthalmoscope. Now dim the room lights.

4. Hold the ophthalmoscope in your right hand and use your right eye to examine the patient's right eye. Your left hand and left eye should be used to examine the patient's left eye. It may take some practice to become comfortable with this. If you have reduced visual acuity in one eye it will be necessary to use your better seeing eye to evaluate both the patient's eyes. This will take some practice to avoid bumping the patient's nose.

5. Instruct the patient to look at a point in the room such that his or her gaze is directed superiorly and approximately 15° temporally. Subsequently, direct the patient to look in different positions of gaze to obtain a better view of the peripheral fundus.

6. Place the top of the ophthalmoscope against your brow. You should now be able to view through the aperture. Rotate the ophthalmoscope handle approximately 10° to 20° nasally from the vertical to avoid the patient's nose. Both of your eyes should be kept open to relax your accommodation. You can now rotate the ophthalmoscope handle to move the beam laterally and vertically.

7. Move closer to the patient until the anterior segment of the eye is in focus (at approximately 12 cm). Now observe the clarity of the media. Opacities will appear as dark areas against a bright red background (the red reflex; see Figure 5.5 below). You can judge the location of the opacity by using the principle of parallax motion. Choose a point of focus, e.g. the iris. If the opacity is **A**nterior to the iris, '**A**gainst' motion will be observed when you move the beam. If the opacity is posterior to the iris, 'with' motion will be observed when you move

result in increased magnification, which is not always desirable. Also, when high amounts of astigmatism or ocular media opacity are present, the image is distorted or degraded.

The other techniques that can be performed to view the fundus are monocular indirect ophthalmoscopy, binocular indirect ophthalmoscopy and fundus biomicroscopy. Table 5.1 compares the optical and observational characteristics with different types of fundus examination.

Table 5.1 Optical and observational characteristics of various fundus examination techniques

Instrument	Image	Stereopsis	Field of view	Magnification	Extent of fundus visible*
Opthalmoscope					
Direct	Erect	No	$\approx 5°$[‡]	$15\times$[‡]	To equator
Monocular indirect	Erect	No	$\approx 12°$	$5\times$	Beyond equator
Binocular indirect					
(50 mm, 20 D lens)	Reversed and inverted	Yes	$\approx 46°$[†]	$3\times$[†]	Entire retinal surface
Volk 60 D	Reversed and inverted	Yes	$67°$**	$17\times$[§]	Beyond equator
Volk 78 D	Reversed and inverted	Yes	$73°$**	$14\times$[§]	Beyond equator
Volk 90 D	Reversed and inverted	Yes	$69°$**	$12\times$[§]	Beyond equator
Volk SuperField NC	Reversed and inverted	Yes	$120°$**	$11\times$[§]	Beyond equator
Volk SuperPupil NC	Reversed and inverted	Yes	$120°$**	$11\times$[§]	Beyond equator

*Through a dilated pupil, with movement of the eye. [†]Varies with condensing lens power. [‡]Varies with refractive error. [§]Using 16× magnification on the slit lamp. **Manufacturer's claims. The slit lamp limits the field of view, therefore the instrument must be moved to observe this extent of the fundus.

the beam. If you note that the opacity is anterior (e.g. on the cornea) ask the patient to blink. If the opacity moves, it is floating in the tears (e.g. mucus or debris). If it does not move it is a true corneal opacity (e.g. scar, dystrophy). Anterior segment abnormalities should be assessed in more detail using a slit-lamp biomicroscope. Move your head laterally and vertically to ensure that all aspects of the crystalline lens have been observed. The patient can change the position of his or her gaze to facilitate this view.

8. Now, move in closer to the patient while decreasing the dioptric power of the focusing lens as you move closer. By doing this, opacities in the vitreous may be observed, such as floaters, cells, hemorrhages, asteroid bodies, etc. If you ask the patient to look up and down, floaters may become visible as they cross the pupil.

9. You should now be as close as possible to the patient without touching the patient's eye. This is very important as the farther away you are from the patient, the smaller the field of view you will obtain. If you are viewing 15° temporally from the patient's line of sight, the disc or retinal vessels should now be in view. If both you and the patient are emmetropic and your accommodation is relaxed, the dioptric value of the lens wheel should be close to zero. If you and/or the patient is uncorrected and ametropic, the lens power necessary to focus on the fundus (i.e. the power in the lens wheel) will be the sum of the refractive errors and your accommodative state. Some practitioners use this as a quick estimation of the patient's spherical refractive state.

10. If you do not see the disc right away but can focus on the vessels, follow the vessels backwards towards the disc. The bifurcation of the vessels forms a 'V' and this will point in the direction you should move to get to the disc.

11. Once you see the disc, focus it clearly using the lens wheel. Bracketing several lens positions may be required before deciding on the optimal focus. Now note the size, shape, colour and margins of the disc. Also, determine if the disc is tilted. The size, shape, location, slope and relative depth of the physiological cupping should be observed. Note the height and width of the physiological cupping as the vertical and horizontal cup-to-disc ratio (see Figure 5.17). The cup margins should be determined by kinking of the vessels as they pass over the margin. Do not assess the cup as the area of pallor, as often the cup extends beyond this area. In deep cupping, the bottom of the cup will focus with less plus than the neuroretinal rim tissue and it can appear grey with central mottling (the lamina cribrosa). Slight parallax movements may help in determining the cup. For a more accurate assessment of the cup, a stereoscopic view is necessary (see fundus biomicroscopy).

12. Evaluate the retinal vasculature. Examine the vessels in a clockwise sequence starting with the superior nasal vessels in the right eye and the superior temporal vessels in the left eye. The major vessels are followed from the disc as far into the periphery as it is possible to see. You should note the vessel diameter, shape (tortuosity), colour,

margins, and the appearance of the arteriovenous crossings (see Figure 5.6 below). The width of the vessels is usually recorded as a ratio of the arteriolar width to the venolar width (A/V ratio) after the second bifurcation (see Recording below).

13. Examine the retinal periphery. Have the patient look into various positions of gaze (up, right, down and left) while systematically sweeping across the retina with a moderately wide beam of light. It is important to be careful, as moderately large abnormalities can be missed easily due to the direct ophthalmoscope's high magnification and narrow field of view. When the patient is looking down it will be necessary to gently hold up the upper lid to view the inferior retina. All abnormalities detected should be assessed in terms of their size, shape, location, colour and depth. The size and location are measured in terms of disc diameters (DD). The location of the abnormality is referenced to the disc and the position is recorded in terms of the clock position relative to the disc (see Figure 5.18). Using a slit may be helpful in determining the elevation of a lesion. If the lesion is elevated, a deviation in the slit will be noted, although elevated lesions should be evaluated using indirect ophthalmoscopy with a stereoscopic view.

14. Finally, evaluate the macula. This observation is performed at the end so that the patient has a chance to adapt to the light; however many patients still find the light uncomfortably bright, therefore dimming the illumination may be required to get an adequate view of the macula. The macula is located slightly below centre and approximately 2 DD temporal to the disc. You can either move the light in this direction or ask the patient to look directly into the light. You will often note a bright reflection from the cornea which obscures the view of the macula. This can be minimised by decreasing the size of the light beam, changing the shape of the light beam (a half moon shape is available with some ophthalmoscopes) or changing your angle of observation. The normal macular pigment and the foveal reflex should be observed. Abnormalities should be assessed in terms of their size, shape, location, colour and depth.

The reticule can be used to determine the presence of eccentric fixation. Ask the patient to look into the centre of the pattern. If the foveal reflex is in the centre of the pattern the patient does not have eccentric fixation. If the reflex is off the centre of the pattern, the amount and direction of eccentric fixation can be measured by comparing the location of the foveal reflex with the location of the rings of the concentric pattern.

Recording

1. Media: correctly identify opacities in the media and record them on a diagram, e.g. for a cataract the location, shape and severity should be clearly recorded (Figure 5.5).
2. Disc: record the width and height of the physiological cupping of the disc as a decimal fraction (see Figure 5.17). The disc is considered one

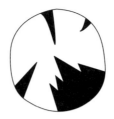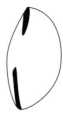

Figure 5.5 Diagram used to record the presence, size and type of cataract after ophthalmoscopic and/or slit lamp examination.

unit and the cup is therefore a fraction of that unit. This should be recorded to ±0.05 accuracy, e.g. 0.60 horizontally and 0.65 vertically. If a reticule is available on the ophthalmoscope, it can make this judgment somewhat easier. The vertical cup-to-disc ratio is of greater significance clinically.

Draw the shape, size and location of the physiological cupping on a diagram of the disc. Include a horizontal cross section of the cupping, showing the depth and shape, and a vertical one if necessary. In the same diagram include all anomalies/abnormalities of the disc, e.g. crescents, papilloedema, tilting, drusen, etc. Note the presence of the lamina cribrosa and if the pores are round or irregular and elongated. Note the presence of spontaneous venous pulsation as well as the colour of the optic nerve head.

3. Vessels: assess the size of the vessels after the second bifurcation from the disc. Compare the relative width of the arteries and veins. It is important to make sure that you are assessing comparable sections of each vessel. This is usually recorded in terms of a ratio, e.g. 2/3. The arterio-venous crossings should be assessed and the presence of abnormalities such as nipping or right angle crossings should be recorded (Figure 5.6). The course of the vessels should be recorded in terms of their tortuosity. If no abnormalities are detected, record 'No abnormalities detected' (NAD), or 'negative' or something equivalent.

4. Fundus: draw the presence of any or all abnormalities/anomalies on a fundus diagram. Do this as accurately as possible, avoiding exaggerations. Note the size, shape, location, colour and depth of the finding (abnormality/anomaly). If you can correctly identify the anomaly, the diagram need only represent the anomaly and be labelled with the diagnosis and location.

The size of a lesion and its location with respect to the disc is usually specified in disc diameters (DD). For example, the lesion may be 2 DD × 1 DD wide. It may be located 4 DD at 4 o'clock from the disc. Record this on the diagram (see Figure 5.18). Describe the general appearance of the fundus, e.g. tessellated, darkly pigmented, blond, etc.

5. Macula: record the presence or absence of a foveal reflex. Any anomalies should be recorded as described for fundus anomalies

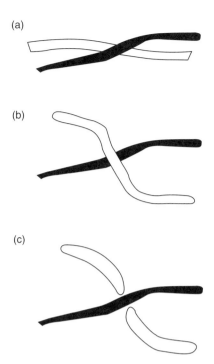

(a)

(b)

(c)

Figure 5.6 (a) A normal artery:vein oblique crossing. (b) A change in direction of a vein to give a 90° crossing over an artery. (c) 'Banking' or 'nipping' of a vein by an artery.

(e.g. drusen, pigmentation changes, haemorrhages, subfoveal neovascular membranes, oedema, etc.).

Interpretation

Normally, the media should be free of any opacities. Vitreous detachment and nuclear sclerosis of the crystalline lens are expected with age. The disc should have a pink rim of tissue surrounding the physiological cupping. The physiological cup-to-disc ratio should be less than 0.60. The arterioles and venuoles should have a smooth course and cross at oblique angles without nipping. The A/V ratio is usually 3/4 or 2/3. Some crossing changes, narrowing of the vessels and colour changes are expected with age. A foveal reflex is usually seen until the end of the third decade. The absence of a foveal reflex in the fifth decade is not abnormal. The fundus should be free of haemorrhages, exudates, and pigmentary disturbances. Occasional naevi and a tessellated fundus represent normal pigmentation. The retina should be attached at all locations. All anomalies/abnormalities noted should be correctly identified as a normal variation or a disease state, and correct management must then be instituted.

Most common errors

1. Assuming that the periphery has been evaluated adequately with a direct ophthalmoscope and a natural pupil.
2. Not getting close enough to the patient when performing the technique.
3. Grading the A/V ratio and crossing changes before the second bifurcation of the vessels.
4. Assuming that any optic disc cupping has been evaluated adequately with the direct ophthalmoscope's non-stereoscopic view.
5. Exaggerating the anomaly in the drawing such that the drawing does not represent the severity or size of the observed condition.

Further reading

Havener, W. (1984). *Synopsis of Ophthalmology*. C.V. Mosby, St. Louis, Missouri
Kanski, J.J. (1989). *Clinical Ophthalmology*. Butterworth–Heinemann, Oxford, UK

Central visual field screening

Background

Perimetry enables the assessment of visual function throughout the visual field, the detection and quantification of damage along the visual pathway, and the monitoring of disease progression. Central visual field screening can be considered part of a routine eye examination for asymptomatic and risk free patients, although new fast, interactive thresholding algorithms may soon supersede such screening techniques (e.g. SITA, TOP). Central screening should *never* be considered for patients exhibiting risk factors for glaucoma, neurologic disease, certain types of retinal disease or symptomatic patients (see Central field quantification below). Similarly, it should never be used to follow the progression of a disease. If defects are suspected following screening then central field quantification should be performed.

Recommended test: Automated perimeter providing a suprathreshold central field screening program, such as the Henson 3200

Rationale

Automated perimetry permits the standardisation of the testing procedure in addition to providing interpretative analysis of the results. Most automated perimeters use static target presentation in which small, stationary targets of variable brightness or size are presented for a fixed time against a calibrated background. Screening strategies sample the visual field at a suprathreshold level, in order to detect advanced defects rapidly. Automated perimetry can be performed by trained clinical assistants. The Henson 3200 was chosen as the recommended procedure because it is the most widely used in the UK at present. By using a multiple stimulus presentation and suprathreshold brightness, the screening is very quick. The multiple stimulus suprathreshold program tests 26 points within the central 25 degree visual field using eight presentations of between two and four points. A threshold value is first determined (the level at which the light can just be detected) at several mid-peripheral points around the 10 degree isopter, and the expected threshold values for the entire visual field are extrapolated. All target locations are then tested at 5 dB brighter than these values (5 dB suprathreshold). If any point is repeatedly missed, the program can be extended to screen 68 or 136 points in the central field. Typical test duration is between 2 and 4 min. The Henson 3200 provides a threshold strategy to assess more accurately any field defects detected using the suprathreshold screening program. The more expensive and less widely available Humphrey visual field analyser and Henson 4000 also provide suprathreshold and threshold assessments and are otherwise preferred as they can assess the 30–60 degree field and provide a facility to monitor the patient's eye position and fixation (see Central visual field quantification below).

Procedure

1. Explain the test and the reasons for performing the assessment to the patient.
2. Turn on the instrument (in this case the Henson 3200).
3. Seat the patient at the perimeter and adjust the height of the instrument and position of the chin rest to ensure patient comfort.
4. Select F1: 'Multiple stimulus suprathreshold' from the main menu.
5. Occlude the left eye and place any appropriate correction for a 33 cm working distance into the lens holder and position before the right eye. Best sphere should be used for any cylinder less than 1.50 D. Full aperture lenses should always be used.
6. Adjust the chin rest for the right eye, and place the patient's head in the rests.
7. Ensure that the vertex distance of the trial lens is adjusted appropriately.
8. Explain that a number of small lights will be flashed on the screen in front of the patient and that he or she should indicate to you how many are seen. Ask the patient to look at the central red light in front of him or her, and indicate the importance of doing so throughout the test. Explain that the patient will see the flashed lights 'out of the corner of the eyes'.

The computer screen provides instructions to guide you through the rest of the examination.

9. First, you must estimate the patient's threshold. The target presentations are set at a bright level and subsequently lowered until none can be seen. One step above this level is taken as threshold. Press the PRESENT button and ask the patient how many flashes of light he or she saw. If the patient saw none, press the ↑ button; if one or more, press the ↓ button. The computer will repeat this procedure until there have been two 'none' responses (and two ↑ button presses).
10. The program will then set the targets at 5 dB above this threshold level in order to screen for a field defect at a suprathreshold level.
11. The program then presents eight stimuli of between two and four points. Press the PRESENT button. If the patient correctly determines the number of targets presented, press the → button to proceed to the

next presentation and press the PRESENT button once again. Continue in this way for all eight presentations or until a target is missed.

12. If a target is missed, present again. If the patient incorrectly identifies the number of targets for a second time, ask the patient to describe the position of the seen targets. They are best described using the positions of the hours on a clock.

13. The targets will be described on the computer screen as A, B, C or D. Press the button which describes the target(s) missed. Then press the PRESENT button again and repeat the procedure.

14. If the same target(s) were missed again, then the computer suggests that you extend the screening program. Press F2 (EXTEND). This extends the screening program to 68 points. The computer screen now also contains a dial which indicates whether the field is normal, suspect or defective.

15. Once you have completed screening the 68 points, reassess any points missed at higher suprathreshold values. Return to the presentation where a target or targets were missed using the → button and increase the intensity of the presentation to 8 dB above threshold by pressing the ↑ button. Present the target at this intensity level. If it is missed at this level, increase the intensity to 12 dB above threshold by again pressing the ↑ button, and present again.

16. If the screening program indicates that the field is suspect or defective, then press F3 (PRINT/SAVE). You will then be asked to input the patient's details and can save the field information on disk and/or request a printout.

Recording

If no errors are made on the eight initial presentations or if the Henson indicates the field is normal on the extended program, then record 'Henson field screener: NAD (suprathreshold level)', e.g. Henson field screener: NAD 2.6 R and L. Figure 5.7 shows the printout of a normal field result.

If there is a field defect, then print the fields of both eyes, attach to the record card and perform a full threshold field.

Interpretation

Any visual field defect is interpreted by the program, which indicates whether it is normal, suspicious or a field defect. The program considers the number, depth and clustering properties of any missed targets when interpreting the field defect. If the program indicates that there is a field defect, there is a 0.1% chance that the field defect is from a patient with a normal field and is due to chance.

The printout of the visual field indicates whether a point was seen at the 5 dB suprathreshold level (▌), or was missed at the 5 dB, 8 dB or 12 dB suprathreshold level:

5 dB ◯   8 dB ◗   12 dB ●

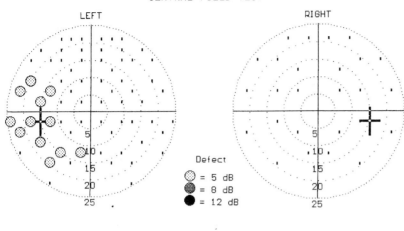

SURNAME.......   FIRST NAME....

BIRTH DATE....   NUMBER.......

MULTIPLE STIM SUPRA-THRESH

CENTRAL FIELD TEST

LEFT   RIGHT

Defect

⊘ = 5 dB
◍ = 8 dB
● = 12 dB

Missed/Presented = 12/68   Missed/Presented = 0/26

Threshold Sensitivity = 29 dB   Threshold Sensitivity = 30 dB

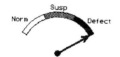

Figure 5.7 The printout of a field result from a Henson 3200 multiple stimulus threshold screening. (Reprinted with permission of Tinsley Medical Instruments).

It is likely that a proportion of early glaucomatous defects detected using central field quantification will be missed using a screening technique of this type.

The program does not present any reliability indices such as the number of fixation losses and the percentage of false positive and false negative errors. This information is provided in the single stimulus screening and full threshold strategies which are available on the Henson 3200, but cannot be obtained when using multiple stimulus presentation. It is left to the clinical judgement of the operator as to whether a field defect could be due to unreliable responses from the patient. Reliability indices are provided with the full threshold strategy, and the reliability of the patient's responses can be quantified using this secondary assessment.

Most common errors

1. Using a suprathreshold screening technique to assess the visual fields of a patient 'at risk' of having a defect (e.g. a suspect primary open-angle glaucoma patient).
2. Aligning the patient poorly (especially as the Henson 3200 has no eye monitoring device).
3. Using an inappropriate refractive correction.
4. Instructing the patient poorly.

Acceptable alternative procedure

Single stimulus suprathreshold measurement is available on most automated perimeters including the Henson 3200 and PRO and others such as the Humphrey VFA, Octopus and Dicon. Single stimulus presentations take slightly longer than multiple stimulus ones for obvious reasons. However, they have the advantage that there is less interpretative interaction by the perimetrist as to the number of targets seen, thus permitting more consistent response criteria. Single stimulus tests also provide information regarding the reliability of the patient, such as the number of fixation losses and the percentage of false positive and false negative errors.

Further reading

Henson, D.B. (1993). *Visual Fields*. Oxford Medical Publications, Oxford, UK
Johnson, C.A. (1997). Perimetry and visual field testing. In *The Ocular Examination: Measurements and Findings* (K. Zadnik, ed.) W.B. Saunders, London

Additional central vision testing

Background

The most common assessment of central visual function is visual acuity measurement. However, this provides just one assessment of central vision and offers little help in differential diagnosis. In addition, some ocular abnormalities can produce little or no reduction in visual acuity, but can produce other changes to central vision, such as centrocaecal scotomas and metamorphopsia.

Recommended test: Amsler charts

Rationale
Although there appears to have been no comparison of the sensitivity of Amsler charts vs.

Procedure

1. Seat the patient comfortably in the examining chair with the appropriate near correction.

2. Position yourself so as to be able to hold the charts at the 30 cm working distance and occlude the non-viewing eye.
3. Keep the room lights on. The method is qualitative and critical light levels are not essential; however, it is useful to be able to reproduce approximate ambient luminance levels.
4. Select the chart for testing:

   Chart 1: the standard chart used in every case. Consists of a 5 mm square, white grid each subtending approximately 1°, on a black background with a central, white fixation target.

   Chart 2: similar to chart 1 but with two diagonal white lines to assist steady fixation in patients with a central scotoma.

   Chart 3: similar to Chart 1 but with a red grid. It has been reported to be useful in the toxic amblyopias and optic neuritis, but is also capable of testing the malingerer when used in conjunction with red and green filters.

   Chart 4: consists of scattered white dots with a central, white fixation target. It is often easier for a patient to define specific or multiple central scotomas.

   Chart 5: consists of white parallel lines only and a central, white fixation point. The orientation of the lines can be adjusted, which can be useful in the detection of metamorphopsia.

   Chart 6: similar to chart 5 but has black lines on a white card with additional lines at 0.5° above and below fixation. This chart is also used to detect metamorphopsia.

   Chart 7: similar to chart 1 but with additional 0.5° squares in the central 8°. This chart is used for detection of subtle macular disease.

5. Instruct the patient to view chart 1 monocularly.
6. Ask the patient if he or she can see the central white dot.
7. Ask the patient if he or she can see all four sides and all four corners of the large square.
8. Ask the patient if any of the small squares within the grid is missing or blurry.
9. Ask the patient if any of the lines that make up the grid appears wavy or distorted.
10. Ask the patient if any part of the grid appears to be flickering, shimmering or coloured.
11. Repeat steps 6 to 10 with any additional chart as deemed appropriate.
12. Record any defects or disturbances on an Amsler recording sheet. It is sometimes useful to have the patient draw the defects on a recording chart (Figure 5.8).

Recording

Record defects or disturbances on an Amsler recording sheet. Always record the eye tested, the date of examination and the patient's name.

central 10° fields measured on an automated perimeter, the Amsler has the advantages that it is much quicker, cheaper and is portable. It is probably the only visual field test that can be used for the home monitoring of progressive, active or recurrent macular disease. In addition, Amsler charts test for metamorphopsia, which is unlikely to be detected by perimeters. The modern Amsler manual consists of seven charts, measuring 10 cm (thus subtending approximately 20° at a working distance of 30 cm). Most patients, other than the very young, will be capable of performing Amsler chart assessment. They are particularly useful for the detection of subtle macula disease such as age-related maculopathy and chloroquine retinopathy.

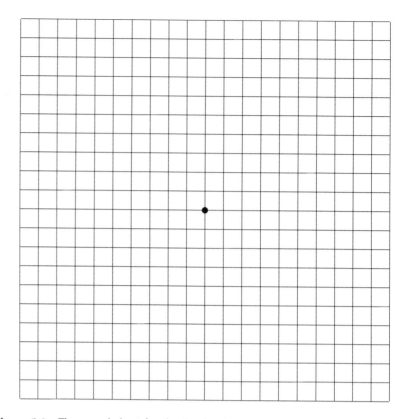

Figure 5.8 The record sheet for the Amsler chart.

Ensure that if no defects are detected, this is recorded clearly in the patient's file, e.g. Amsler charts: NAD R and L.

Interpretation

Metamorphopsia may indicate subtle macular disease. Scotomas indicate more severe retinal or optic nerve disease. The detection of metamorphopsia can be a very sensitive indicator of macular problems. Although this can be advantageous clinically, great care must be taken when choosing the suitability of a patient for the test, particularly if home monitoring is being considered, as it can point out otherwise undetectable problems that subsequently greatly annoy patients.

Most common errors

1. Performing the test binocularly.
2. Using an inappropriate near correction.
3. Using an incorrect working distance.
4. Using the patient's bifocals with a small reading area.
5. Not ensuring that the patient views the central fixation target throughout the test.

Further reading

Patorgis, C.J. (1991). Amsler charts. In *Clinical Procedures in Optometry* (J.B. Eskridge, J.F. Amos and J.D. Bartlett, eds) J.B. Lippincott, Philadelphia, Pennsylvania

Additional acceptable procedure: Photostress recovery time

Procedure

1. Measure distance visual acuity.
2. Ask the patient to remove their spectacles, but keep them in his or her lap so that they can be quickly put back on again.
3. Occlude one eye. Hold your direct ophthalmoscope about 2–3 cm away from the patient's eye. Turn on the light and ask the patient to look directly at the light for exactly 10 sec.
4. After 10 sec, remove the ophthalmoscope, ask the patient to put his or her glasses back on and point to the letters one line larger than the patient's original visual acuity. Ask the patient to read those letters as quickly as he or she can after the after-image has disappeared.
5. Time how long it takes after removal of the bleaching light for the patient to read at least $\frac{2}{3}$ of the letters indicated.
6. Repeat the measurement for the other eye if necessary.

Recording

Record the time taken in seconds to recover to within one line of pre-bleached visual acuity in sec.

Interpretation

It is generally suggested that any PSRT longer than 50 sec is abnormal, and suggests a macular disease rather than optic nerve abnormality. Of course, a normal PSRT depends on the brightness of the light used, and it is best to obtain your own normal values with your own particular technique and instrumentation.

Most common errors

1. Allowing the patient to lose fixation of the bleaching light.
2. Using a direct ophthalmoscope with batteries which are not fully charged.
3. Having the patient wait until the letters are clearly visible rather than just visible.
4. Timing inaccurately.

Rationale

Photostress recovery time (PSRT) is a measurement of the time taken for visual acuity to return to normal levels after the macula is bleached by a bright light. PSRT is dependent purely on the photochemical capability of the macula, and prolonged PSRT can be found with age-related maculopathy (ARM), angiod-streaks, choroideremia, serous retinal detachment, and pigment epithelium retinopathy. PSRT testing is probably most useful clinically in differentiating macular from optic nerve disease as the cause of central vision loss can occasionally be difficult to diagnose due to inconclusive funduscopic findings. As optic nerve disorders do not affect the photochemical processes in the photoreceptors, recovery times remain normal. PSRT may also aid in monitoring the recovery or progression of maculopathies such as early cystoid macular edema, idiopathic central serous chorioretinopathy, and chloroquine or solar burn effects on the macula.

Further reading

Elliott, D.B. (1997). Supplementary clinical tests of vision. In *The Optometric Examination: Measurement and Findings* (K. Zadnik, ed.) W.B. Saunders, London, UK

Central visual field quantification

Background

Threshold automated perimetry is the standard of care for the diagnosis and management of many ocular and neurologic diseases. In particular it plays an invaluable role in the diagnosis and management of the glaucomas. Quantification of the central visual field is not indicated as part of a routine eye examination for asymptomatic and risk-free patients, although new, fast thresholding strategies may make such an approach more feasible. However, such testing should be performed on all patients complaining of symptoms consistent with central field loss, symptomatic neurologic cases, patients with risk factors for glaucoma and patients who have demonstrated possible abnormality using a screening technique (e.g. positive Amsler, confrontation or automated screening test). In addition threshold fields are always required when monitoring a known defect (e.g. should always be included in protocols for co-management of glaucoma). Screening fields test at 5–6 dB above threshold, so that subtle field defects may be missed.

The use of fast thresholding strategies examination (e.g. HFA, SITA, SITAFast, Fastpac and Octopus TOPs and Dynamic Strategy) may be better for some patients, such as the typical elderly glaucoma patient. It has been demonstrated that the decreased accuracy of the fast strategy can be counterbalanced by the reduction of fatigue effects due to the shorter test time. Younger or sprightly patients capable of concentrating for a longer examination time (15 vs. 8 min per eye) can be considered for the full threshold strategy. Most patients other than the very young will be capable, with appropriate instruction, of performing central visual field quantification.

Recommended test

Rationale
The Humphrey Field Analyser (HFA) II is used as an example of a state-of-the-art perimeter capable of performing threshold tests over the central 30° of the visual field, using a single target presentation. Multiple stimulus

Humphrey Field Analyser II or equivalent (e.g. Humphrey Field Analyser model 610 or higher, Henson PRO, Octopus 1-2-3, Octopus 101, Dicon), Central 30-2 threshold program.

The HFA Central 30-2 tests 76 locations over the central 30° in a 6° grid pattern that straddles the horizontal and vertical mid-lines, i.e. targets are located 3° either side of the mid-lines. Equivalent programs can be found on most perimeters. The 24-2 program on the Humphrey could also be used. It only tests the central 25° rather than 30°, but consequently testing time is reduced by 20% and fatigue is reduced.

Procedure

1. Turn on the instrument.
2. The patient should be seated at the perimeter and the height of the instrument and position of the chin rest adjusted to ensure patient comfort.
3. At the 'Main Menu' select 'Central 30-2'.
4. Select the eye to be tested first, and unless otherwise indicated select 'Right'.
5. Enter the patient ID. Let the patient adapt to the bowl luminance while entering the data. Enter as much patient data as possible but always include patient name using the surname first, date of birth (NB this is often formatted as month–day–year) and patient file number if appropriate. It is often useful to enter the prescription lenses used and pupil size. It is also possible to enter diagnostic code, VA, IOP and C:D.
6. Select 'Change Parameters', followed by 'Test Strategy' and ensure 'Fastpac' is selected. If a full threshold strategy is considered appropriate, select 'Full Threshold'.
7. Occlude the left eye, give the patient the response button and place any appropriate correction into the lens holder and position before the right eye. Best sphere should be used for any cylinder less than 1.50 D. Full aperture lenses should always be used.
8. Place the patient's head in the headrest. Explain the test to the patient. Select 'Help Icon' if unsure of patient instruction.
9. Align the patient using the video eye monitor.
10. Ensure that the vertex distance of the trial lens is adjusted appropriately.
11. Select 'Demo' for a naïve patient. Repeat until you are happy that the patient understands the procedure.
12. Select 'Start'.
13. Some models will have a Gaze Monitoring feature. Once initialised select 'Start'.
14. Monitor fixation and encourage the patient throughout the test.
15. *Never* leave the patient unattended.
16. Encourage the patient to rest during the test, particularly if false negative catch trials are noted.
17. Pause the test and re-instruct the patient if catch trials, particularly false positives, are noted.
18. When the test is completed, store the result on disk then select 'Test Other Eye'. Occlude the patient's right eye and align the left eye with the appropriate correction having been placed in the lens holder.
19. When the left eye is completed, store the results on disk and select 'Print' or the print icon.
20. Print all results and return to the 'Main Menu'.

presentation cannot be used to determine thresholds, and single stimulus presentation has the advantage that there is less interpretive interaction by the perimetrist as to the number of targets seen, thus permitting more consistent response criteria. The test is also more suitable for use by support staff as they cannot as easily influence the test result other than by encouraging the patient and monitoring fixation. There are many automated perimeters that are similarly capable of such testing. The Henson PRO is preferred over the Henson 3200 for visual field quantification because it enables patient fixation to be monitored.

Optional/additional testing

Rationale

Macular testing should be performed as an alternate to the central 30-2 program in macula disease and advanced glaucoma. It should also be considered in patients that demonstrate a positive Amsler test. The HFA Central 10-2 tests 68 locations over the central 10° in a 2° grid pattern that straddles the horizontal and vertical mid-lines, i.e. targets are located 1° either side of the mid-lines. Equivalent programs can be found on most perimeters.

Rationale

Peripheral testing should be considered in some neurological cases, occasional retinal and glaucoma cases, when patients report symptoms of poor peripheral vision and when assessing vision standards. The three zone, threshold related, age referenced, screening strategy is adequate for the assessment of peripheral visual function, being equivalent to a three isopter manual kinetic test.

Macular testing

Recommended test: Humphrey Field Analyser II Central 10-2 threshold program or equivalent.

Procedure. The same as central visual field quantification but replace program 30-2 with program 10-2.

Advantages
1. More appropriate for investigation of the central 10°.
2. Higher spatial resolution in the central 10°.

Disadvantage
Only assesses the central 10°.

Peripheral testing

Recommended test: Humphrey Field Analyser II Peripheral 60 screening program or equivalent (e.g. Humphrey Field Analyser I Peripheral 68 screening program).

Procedure
1. Following completion of the 30-2 field select 'Screening' test type from the 'Main Menu'.
2. Select 'Peripheral 60'.
3. Select 'Right'.
4. Select 'Change Parameters'.
5. Select 'Three Zone' test strategy.
6. Select 'Age Reference Level' test mode.
7. Follow steps 7 to 18. No prescription lenses will be used for any patient.
8. When the left eye is completed, store the results on disk.
9. Select 'File Function Icon' from the 'Main Menu' and merge the Central 30-2 and Peripheral 60 files for printing.

Recording

Automated, but it is useful to describe the shape of any defect found and record a subjective opinion of the patient's reliability.

Interpretation

Visual fields should be interpreted with respect to their reliability, as a single field and with respect to change over time.

The reliability indices consist of fixation losses, which should be less than 30%; false positive and false negative catch trials, which should be less than 20%; and short-term fluctuations, which should be within normal limits (not have a reported p-value). False positive errors indicate a 'trigger happy' patient who is responding when no target is presented. False negative errors accumulate when a patient fails to respond to a suprathreshold target at a given location; these are associated with fatigue and/or inattention. Short-term fluctuation is a score of intra-test variability.

The single field analysis includes: the sensitivity level for each point in decibels; an interpolated grey scale display; the total deviation in decibels and probability of each point being normal in a non-interpolated grey scale; the pattern deviation in decibels and probability of each point being normal in a non-interpolated grey-scale; and the glaucoma hemifield analysis.

Total deviation compares the result to an age-matched normal population and states the probability of each point being abnormal on a point-by-point basis.

Pattern deviation compares the result to an age-matched normal population corrected for the overall level of sensitivity for the individual. The probability of any point varying from this level is stated on a point-by-point basis. This enhances the ability to observe mappable scotomata within a generalised depression which may be induced by small pupils or poor media.

A generalised depression will be most easily appreciated by looking for a majority of abnormal points on the total deviation probability chart. Clusters of two or more non-edge points together on the pattern deviation chart ($p < 0.05$) should be considered suspicious. An isolated point within the central $10°$ ($p < 0.05$) should also be considered suspicious. If a cluster of abnormal points exists it should be interpreted with respect to its underlying anatomical correlate and subsequent clinical significance.

The glaucoma hemifield test analyses the relative symmetry of five predefined areas in the superior and inferior field, as well as judging the overall level of sensitivity compared to age-matched normal values. The visual field is then classified as being 'within normal limits', 'outside normal limits', 'borderline' or to have a 'general reduction of sensitivity'.

The global indices are data reduction statistics designed to describe specific characteristics of the glaucomatous visual field. In summary:

- Mean deviation (MD) is a measure of average sensitivity.
- Pattern standard deviation (PSD) is a measure of non-uniformity in the shape of the hill of vision, i.e. is sensitive to early mappable scotoma.
- Short-term fluctuation (SF) is a measure of the intra-test variance.
- Corrected pattern standard deviation (CPSD) is PSD corrected for the SF.

The probability of the global indices being normal is stated on the printout.

Change in the visual field of a single patient over time is best appreciated using the Overview printout. If a glaucomatous defect is being followed, the glaucoma change probability can be considered. In this analysis subsequent fields are compared to the average of two baseline fields and the probability of real glaucomatous change is categorised and illustrated. It is also possible, in the Change Analysis printout, to monitor change in the global indices by linear regression analysis and overall change by means of a box-plot chart.

Most common errors

1. Aligning the patient poorly.
2. Instructing the patient poorly.
3. Using an inappropriate refractive correction.
4. Using an incorrect vertex distance for the trial lenses.
5. Examining the right eye with a left eye program.
6. Failing to encourage and communicate with the patient.
7. Abandoning the patient during the examination.

Further reading

Choplin, N.T. and Edwards, R.P. (1995). *Visual Field Testing with the Humphrey Field Analyzer.* Slack Incorporated, Thorofare, New Jersey

Flanagan, J.G., Buys, Y. and Trope, G.E. (1996). *Automated Perimetry: An Interactive Primer.* Lifelearn Eyecare, Waterloo, Canada

Hodapp, E., Parrish, R.K. II and Anderson, D.R. (1993). *Clinical Decisions in Glaucom.* C.V. Mosby, St. Louis, Missouri

Johnson, C.A. (1997). Perimetry and visual field testing. In *The Ocular Examination: Measurements and Findings* (K. Zadnik, ed.) W.B. Saunders, London, UK

Diagnostic drugs

Notes

1. It should be noted that availability of drugs in the following text has been restricted to those which the optometrist can legally obtain/supply/use. In some cases, therefore, the drugs recommended may not be those which are otherwise recognised as being the drug of choice. This anomaly arises wholly as a result of the limited and somewhat outdated list of drugs which are legally obtainable by the optometrist. A full list of drugs which are obtainable can be found in *The College of Optometrists Formulary* (see references)
2. Some drugs previously listed as being available to optometrists, although useful, have ceased to be commercially obtainable. Drugs such as thymoxamine fall into this category.
3. Storage recommendations for each pharmaceutical can be found within its packaging. In general, a cool darkened room is adequate for most. There are however some diagnostic drugs, such as ophthaine, which need to be refrigerated.
4. Table 5.2 lists the common Latin abbreviations used in ophthalmic prescription writing.

Table 5.2 Common Latin abbreviations used in ophthalmic prescription writing

Latin	Abbreviation	Meaning
Admove	Admov	Apply
Bis in di'e	b.i.d.	Twice a day
Gram	g, gm	Gram
Gutta	gt, Gt	A drop
Hora	h	An hour
Hora somni	h.s.	At bedtime
Nocte	nocte	At night
Per os	p.o.	By mouth
Pro re nata	p.r.n.	When needed
Quaque	q	Each, every
Quaque hora	q.h.	Every hour
Quater in di'e	q.i.d	Four times a day
Recipe	Rx	Take, you take
Signatura	Sig	Write, you write
Sine	s	Without
Solutio	Sol	Solution
Tabella	tab	Tablet
Ter in di'e	t.i.d.	Three times a day
Unguentum	ung	Ointment
Ut dictum	Ut dict	As directed
Unus	i	One
Duo	ii	Two
Tres	iii	Three
Quattour	iv	Four
Quinque	v	Five

Background

In the UK, the use of medicinal products is governed by the Medicines Act 1968, along with a number of statutory instruments.

This legislation places such products into one of the three following groups:

General sales list (GSL)

These are generally products which are can be used relatively safely by members of the public without the need for any supervisory conditions attached to their sale. Thus any retailer can sell such products so long as the premises used for storage are secure.

Pharmacy medicines (P)

The sale of these products must be supervised by a registered pharmacist from premises carrying out business as a retail pharmacy. An optometrist is allowed to supply any eye drop or ointment which is a pharmacy medicine.

Prescription only medicines (PoM)

These are products which are available to the public only according to a medical, dental or veterinary prescription. It is recognised that drugs such as those used for mydriasis, for example, should be available to the optometrist and to this end exemption from the restriction of supply has been granted. A full list of PoMs available to the optometrist can be found in *The College of Optometrists Formulary*.

Through these exemptions, optometrists may supply a patient with certain drugs directly by retail sale or indirectly via a 'signed order' to a pharmacist. The signed order should be written in indelible ink and should include the following information:

1. The optometrist's name and address.
2. Name and address of patient if applicable.
3. The purpose for which the PoM is to be supplied and its name, quantity, pharmaceutical form and strength.
4. Labelling instructions where applicable.
5. An original signature of the optometrist.

The legislation above serves not only to categorise medicines into certain groups but also outlines the circumstances in which optometrists may use drugs. These are:

1. In the course of their professional practice, and
2. In an emergency.

Clearly the above gives some leeway in the optometric use of drugs, since the interpretation of an emergency is left to the discretion of the optometrist who should, obviously, give due regard to the Opticians Act, the GOC rules and the Medicines Act. If an optometrist has previously not considered using any of these drugs and now wishes to do so, then Continuing Education and Training is essential.

A small subsection of the PoM list allows only optometric use rather than supply. The intention here is to prevent such products as topical anaesthetics from being supplied to the patient for analgesia.

In the following text the legal categories of drugs will be referred to as GSL, P or PoM as appropriate. It should be noted that, unless otherwise stated, all PoM drugs are for optometric use and supply.

Rationale

There must be a valid optometric reason for using any diagnostic drug. This rationale must be discussed with the patient before drug instillation so that he or she can provide informed consent to the procedure.

Before selecting a drug the following points should be considered:

1. Indications.
2. Contraindications (taking into account the type of drug to be used, its mechanism of action and its likely effect on an individual patient).
3. Dosage (i.e. concentration and number of drops).
4. Potential side effects with normally used dosage.
5. Appropriate follow-up procedures and/or emergency care should any untoward reactions or sequelae occur. An unwanted reaction such as a rise in intraocular

pressure (IOP) can develop some hours later. The patient should be told who to contact in case of an emergency.

After selecting the appropriate drug, the following should be performed:

1. The expiry date on bottle checked .
2. The container should be checked for discoloration and/or precipitates.

If the expiration date has passed, or if there are precipitates, discoloration or other signs of contamination, the suspect container should be discarded and a new one obtained.

Procedure

Pre-instillation assessment

1. Case history. It should be determined whether the patient or subject has any known hypersensitivity to the diagnostic agent (or any of the ingredients in the pharmaceutical such as any of its preservatives). Inquire about all allergies to medications or eye drops.

   Determine whether the patient has any systemic disease, ocular disease or general systemic condition that could be aggravated by the use of a diagnostic drug. For example, patients with severe cardiovascular disease or hypertension should not be given phenylephrine eye drops.
2. Visual acuity. Visual acuity must always be measured and recorded before any procedure is carried out on the patient.
3. Biomicroscope examination. The corneal integrity should be checked before any drops are instilled and after any procedure involving the cornea. Assessment and estimation of the anterior chamber angle should be performed before using any drug which has mydriatic or cycloplegic effects. A van Herick assessment may not be possible with some patients such as young children and a pen light shadow assessment of the angle should be used (see Anterior chamber angle depth estimation).
4. Tonometry. Tonometry should be performed before the use of a mydriatic or cycloplegic. Patients considered to be at risk from adverse reactions should be advised what to do if any adverse reaction occurs once they have left your care (i.e. ensure that they know who to contact and that they are knowledgeable of the procedures which were carried out).

Drug instillation

1. Carefully identify any drops before instillation by checking the brand name, ingredients, expiration date, discoloration, precipitates.
2. Before the instillation record the drug type (preferably by its brand name) and dosage (i.e. concentration and number of drops used in each eye). The use of the *brand* name is useful since it uniquely identifies the particular preparation which has been used. Different

brands may well have different preservatives or other non-active ingredients.

3. The patient must be seated in a fixed chair with a proper back support and arm rests. There is a chance that upon instillation, the patient (especially a child) will move violently. Therefore under no circumstances should a stool or a chair on casters be used.

4. Check the container of diagnostic drug again for its identity and remove the cap in preparation for drug instillation. If a dropper bottle is being used, do not place the dropper cap on any surface in such a way as to risk contaminating the inside of the bottle cap. It is best if you hold it in your hand.

5. Have the patient tilt his or her head backwards with the chin raised slightly.

6. Direct the patient's gaze upwards.

7. Gently pull down the lower lid or pull it forward slightly to form a pouch.

8. Instil a drop or drops into the temporal side of the pouch. Avoid touching the eyelashes, lids or conjunctiva with the dropper tip. Gently release the lower lid.

9. In the case of ointment, gently squeeze a 1.5 cm ribbon of ointment inside the lower fornix. Ointments, if available, are sometimes preferred to drops because:

   (a) Less can be applied therefore there is less chance of systemic absorption.
   (b) They are more comfortable.
   (c) They are easier to apply even to children.

10. Ask the patient to look downward and gently release the upper lid over the eye.

11. Press firmly over the lacrimal sac (just medial to the inner canthus) for at least 10 sec. This technique of nasolacrimal occlusion ensures that any excess drug which may otherwise enter the nasolacrimal duct is prevented from doing so. Thus, systemic absorption is kept to absolute minimum and the maximum amount of drug is absorbed at the appropriate site. Note that nasolacrimal occlusion is not required when an ointment is used. Wipe any excess drops/ointment away from the eye with a tissue.

12. If two drops are to be used, wait at least 3 min between drops. Instilling two drops consecutively without this wait would overfill the lacrimal lake and the drug would overspill onto the cheek, thereby negating the theoretical enhanced effect of applying more drug.

13. Return the cap to the bottle (and screw on securely) or dispose of single dose products such as Minims® (Chauvin) in an appropriate waste bin. Single dose containers are designed to be used once and discarded. Repeated instillations on different patients with single dose products increases the chance of container contamination since they are normally preservative free. In addition, the drop size squeezed from such containers reduces with repeated instillations, leading to poorer patient response than anticipated.

14. In the case of an anaesthetic, wait 1 min before initiating the procedure(s) to allow time for the drug to take effect.
15. In the case of mydriatics/cycloplegics, make a note of the time of instillation and instruct the patient that it will take approximately 20–45 min (depending on the choice of drug and the individual patient response) for dilation to occur or effective cycloplegia to be achieved.
16. If dilation has not obviously commenced after 15 min, and only one drop of mydriatic (or cycloplegic) has been used, instil a second drop and record this on the patient record.
17. At the conclusion of the examination, record any untoward signs (or symptoms) that occurred during the procedures. Monitor the patient until you are satisfied that there are no serious sequelae to the instillation of the diagnostic agent.

Topical anaesthetics

Indications

1. Applanation tonometry.
2. Gonioscopy.
3. Vitreous lens or fundus lens procedures.
4. Examination of corneal abrasions.
5. To permit removal of foreign bodies.
6. Ultrasonography.

Contraindications

Known allergy to a particular topical anaesthetic or any of the ingredients in the pharmaceutical.

Precautions

1. One or two drops of anaesthetic is all that is usually necessary for a routine examination. Avoid using further drops without careful consideration. If more fluorescein is required and you have used a fluorescein/anaesthetic, use a fluorescein strip rather than adding an additional drop of the combination.
2. Caution patients about rubbing their eyes for at least 30 min after drug instillation in view of the danger of causing an inadvertent corneal abrasion.

Adverse effects

1. Sloughing of the corneal epithelium may occur within a period of 15 min following the instillation of topical anaesthetic in sensitive individuals. Your patient will probably complain of some ocular discomfort (irritation, some pain, enhanced lacrimation and some mild

hyperaemia or injection). Biomicroscope examination will reveal a roughened corneal surface that stains diffusely with fluorescein. Once the anaesthetic has worn off, the patient may experience some blur along with mild or moderate ocular pain. Further anaesthetic should not be used. There is no need for further treatment or for keeping the patient in the office. Aspirin, or its equivalent, will help relieve discomfort but do not recommend aspirin to patients who are known to be allergic to aspirin or related drugs, or have history of gastro-intestinal disturbances.

Patients should be reassured that their eyes will return to normal over the next 24 hours and they should again be reminded of the importance of not rubbing their eyes during this period. 'Eyewhiteners' or contact lenses should not be used during this period. Arrange to check the patient to ensure that the corneas have cleared.

2. There is always a possibility that a patient may faint during any procedure. This is usually caused by undue apprehension about the procedure being performed. When a patient feels faint, loss of consciousness may be averted if the person lies flat or sits with the head bent low. Cold water applied to the back of the neck may help. It is important to anticipate and prevent any injurious fall. Full consciousness should gradually return after several minutes. Whenever a patient loses consciousness remember the ABCs of first aid: check the airways (A), breathing (B) and circulation (C) pulse. Be prepared to administer cardiopulmonary resuscitation (CPR) if necessary.

Available topical ocular anaesthetics (all PoM use only):

Amethocaine hydrochloride 0.5% and 1% (generic) 10 ml bottles and 0.5% and 1% Minims® (Chauvin).
Lignocaine hydrochloride 4.0%, fluorescein sodium BP 0.25% – Minims.
Benoxinate hydrochloride 0.4% – Minims.
Proxymetacaine hydrochloride 0.5% – Ophthaine (Squibb) 15 ml bottles.

Recommended anaesthetics

Most topical anaesthetics give adequate depth of anaesthesia for the above indications and their times of onset are similar at around a minute. Amethocaine tends to be more toxic to the cornea and hence is now used rarely for supplementary diagnostic procedures. Benoxinate hydrochloride 0.4% tends to be the drug of choice since it has a tendency to sting less than other preparations. It is commercially available in Minims single dose form only and this can be expensive if used routinely, in contact tonometry for example. Proxymetacaine or proparacaine hydrochloride as Ophthaine is a useful multidose container alternative. It should be noted that because of the pH dependency of fluorescence of sodium fluorescein, it is not good practice to wet a fluorescein strip with an anaesthetic as this will markedly reduce the fluorescence. Lignocaine hydrochloride as Minims lignocaine 4% combined with fluorescein 0.25% can be a convenient way of instilling this combination for contact tonometry, but it does tend to sting somewhat and there is a tendency for too much fluorescein to be instilled, which can make interpretation of Goldmann rings difficult.

Dosage regimen

i Gt. BE

If a patient either reports persisting ocular sensitivity, a previous experience with poor anaesthetic effect, or when you suspect continued sensitivity after a single drop, two drops can be used safely and effectively. At least 3 min should be allowed to elapse between each drop instillation.

Mydriatics

Indications

A fundus and media examination through a dilated pupil should be considered if the following conditions present:

1. When there is a reduction in visual acuity.
2. When there is difficulty in obtaining an adequate view of the posterior fundus. In particular, this indicates the need for a dilated fundus examination prior to any referral for cataract surgery.
3. For the differential diagnosis of any media or fundus abnormalities. In such cases a stereoscopic view of the fundus and/or media is preferred to make a more certain diagnosis.
4. In the routine examination of the diabetic patient so as to ascertain the presence and degree of diabetic retinopathy, and particularly macular oedema, which is difficult to spot with direct ophthalmoscopy through an undilated pupil.
5. In any patient with primary open angle glaucoma (POAG) or 'at risk' of having the disease, e.g. high IOPs, different IOPs in the two eyes, suspicious discs, family history of POAG or a central visual field defect. The disc can be assessed properly only in a stereoscopic view.
6. In any patient 'at risk' of having a retinal detachment, e.g. symptoms such as photopsia, 'spots', 'veils', or 'shadows'; myopia of a degree greater than 4 D or in any eye showing myopic degeneration; a family history of retinal detachment; a previous retinal detachment in either eye or history of ocular trauma.
7. In any patient with aphakia or pseudophakia (apart from iris clip intraocular lenses in which mydriasis is contraindicated due to the danger of the lens becoming dislodged) in order to eliminate the presence of surgical complications, including retinal detachment or cystoid macular oedema.
8. In any patient suspected of having macular oedema and similar diseases which are difficult to spot with direct ophthalmoscopy through an undilated pupil, e.g. symptoms of distorted vision, sudden loss of vision, monocular increase in hyperopia, etc.
9. For fundus, lens or vitreous photography.

10. Monocular patients.

The ideal situation would be to examine all first time patients stereoscopically through a dilated pupil and at regular intervals subsequently.

Contraindications

1. The known or suspected presence of angle closure glaucoma or the suspected predisposition to angle closure glaucoma (i.e. angles capable of closing under the influence of a mydriatic or cycloplegic). A cornea/anterior chamber ratio of 1 : 0.25 (van Herick grade II) or less indicates an 'at risk' eye and gonioscopy should be performed to ensure that dilation is safe.
2. Known hypersensitivity to the mydriatic or cycloplegic or other components of these pharmaceuticals.
3. Presence of an iris-supported intraocular iris implant.
4. Subluxated crystalline lens or dislocated intraocular lens implant.
5. The patient's activities in the period immediately following the use of these agents require clear near and distance vision (e.g. driving, operating heavy machinery).
6. Phenylephrine 10% should not be used. Phenylephrine 2.5% should be used with caution if:

    (a) the patient is a hypertensive or has cardiac disease.
    (b) the patient is under medication with monoamine oxidase inhibitors, e.g. phenelzine (Nardil), tranylcypromine (Parnate), or trycyclic antidepressants, e.g. nortriptyline (Aventyl), imipramine (Tofranil), trimipramine (Surmontil). See Adverse effects below.

Adverse effects

1. Photophobia may be experienced in many individuals, simply as a result of the pupillary dilation.
2. Fainting or mild palpitation (racing of the heart). As with the instillation of topical ocular anaesthetics, some patients may be predisposed to a 'fright' reaction simply because they are nervous about the procedure.
3. It should be noted that angle closure is very rarely induced by the instillation of a mydriatic/cycloplegic agent especially if the appropriate precautions are followed before drug instillation. (See Therapeutics section in Chapter 6 for details to deal with closed angle glaucoma.)
4. Excessive topical doses of phenylephrine (multiple drops of 2.5% or one or more drops of 10%) can cause a systemic hypertensive crisis in predisposed individuals receiving monoamine oxidase inhibitors or tricylic antidepressant drugs. If such an event occurs, the patient will complain of sudden, severe, occipital headache, dizziness, and weakness. The patient should be reclined and the examiner should

watch for possible cardiac arrest. The examiner should be prepared to administer CPR if necessary.

Available mydriatic agents

Tropicamide hydrochloride (PoM) 0.5% and 1.0% – Minims (Chauvin); Mydriacyl (Alcon) 5 ml bottles.
Phenylephrine hydrochloride (P) 2.5% and 10% – Minims. Note that the 10% concentration gives no more mydriasis than the 2.5% but gives significantly increased risk of cardio-vascular adverse effects and therefore its use cannot normally be justified.

Recommended mydriatics and suggested dosage regimens

1. Tropicamide 0.5%. Two drops each eye, with each drop being separated by at least 3 min.
2. Tropicamide 1.0%. One drop may be sufficient for patients with blue irides but two drops for patients with brown irides.
3. Some patients respond less well than others and occasionally a second drop (particularly when the 0.5% concentration has been used) is necessary. In general, patients with lighter irides (e.g. blue) will respond quicker and to a greater degree than those patients with dark irides. The instillation of two drops of a lower concentration is generally considered more efficacious than a single instillation of a higher concentration since, ultimately, more of the drug is absorbed by the 'two drop with a wait' regimen.
4. A combination drug procedure may be used when greater dilation is required, such as when using binocular indirect ophthalmoscopy and when fundus, lens or vitreous photography is required. In this procedure, one drop of phenylephrine 2.5% is instilled in each eye and then, 3 min later, one drop of tropicamide 0.5% (or 1%) is instilled in each eye. Phenylephrine is a poor mydriatic on its own as it leaves the innervation of the sphincter intact and pupil responses to light are therefore retained.
5. A topical ocular anaesthetic can be used before the instillation of a mydriatic or cycloplegic agent (one may have been used for contact tonometry). The anaesthetic, as well as reducing possible discomfort, can reduce lacrimation and thus reduce drug wash-out for subsequently instilled drugs. It has also been suggested that the mildly toxic effects of a topical anaesthetic on the cornea opens up the intracellular spaces and aids penetration of other drugs. The above factors result in an enhanced effect of mydriatics or cycloplegic. After instillation of the anaesthetic, wait at least 3 min before instilling the mydriatic/cycloplegic.

Cycloplegics

Indications

1. Patients with pseudomyopia or latent hyperopia.
2. Strabismus patients with a suspected accommodative component.
3. When needed to control accommodation, examples of which could be:

    (a) In the very young child.
    (b) In patients whose subjective refraction is variable.
    (c) In young myopes with significant esophoria.
    (d) In young patients who have symptoms but apparently no significant refractive error.

Contraindications

1. Narrow-angle glaucoma or narrow angles predisposed to closure (see section on mydriatics above). This is less likely to occur with cycloplegics, which are generally used on a much younger population than mydriatics. The anterior angle is wider in children and young adults and gets smaller throughout adulthood due to the increase in size of the lens.
2. Known hypersensitivity to a specific cycloplegic and/or its components.

Adverse effects

1. Blurred vision resulting from cycloplegia.
2. Photophobia due to mydriasis.
3. All these drugs (with the exception of tropicamide, for which no serious adverse effects have been recorded) can give rise to systemic effects such as altered mental states and increased heart rates.
4. Rarely, psychotic reactions have been reported in infants, children and teenagers following the use of cyclopentolate. It is possible that such reactions could occur when using cyclopentolate 0.5% or 1%. In such reactions, the patient appears disorientated and may hallucinate. Recovery is spontaneous after 1 or 2 hours, without any treatment being required.
5. Atropine is highly toxic. If this drug is used, a patient instruction sheet is needed, e.g.

    (a) Wash hands before and after instillation.
    (b) Squeeze out about a grape-pip size amount and apply inside the lower eyelid of both eyes.
    (c) Apply twice a day. The last application should be on the night before the appointment.
    (d) Excess ointment should be removed with cotton wool and burned.
    (e) After the 3-day application the tube should be burned.

(f) Other people should not use the ointment.
(g) Keep the drug under lock and key.
(h) Stop using the drug if an allergic reaction occurs.
(i) It is often easier to instil the drug if the child is asleep.

You should also be aware of the systemic effects of atropine poisoning which are as follows: dry mouth, tachycardia, headache, fever, irregular pulse, mental aberration, respiratory depression, coma, death. Atropine is a potentially dangerous drug especially in young children. Several instances of toxic side effects from atropine installation have been reported. These are more likely with:

(a) The use of drops instead of ointment.
(b) Blond children.
(c) Down's syndrome children.
(d) Children with spastic paralyses.
(e) Patients with renal impairment.

Other than toxic systemic effects the ocular adverse effects are mainly allergic responses, including red, crusty flaking skin of the eyelids and injected bulbar conjunctiva. Prolonged use may cause follicular conjunctivitis.

Available cycloplegic agents

In relative order of use:

1. Cyclopentolate (PoM) 0.5% and 1%, Minims (Chauvin), Mydrilate (Boehinger Ingelheim) 5 ml bottles.
2. Tropicamide (PoM) 1% Minims, Mydriacyl (Alcon) 5 ml bottles.
3. Atropine (PoM) 1% Minims, Isopto Atropine (Alcon), 1% and 0.5% atropine sulphate ointment (generic).
4. Homatropine (PoM) 1% and 2% (generic), 1% Minims.

Suggested dosage regimen and clinical use of cycloplegics

As with the use of mydriatic, the instillation of cycloplegic agents may be preceded by instillation of a topical anaesthetic. At least 3 min must elapse before proceeding with instillation of the cycloplegic drug.

Cyclopentolate
Age < 12 years i Gt. 1.0%
Age > 12 years i Gt. 0.5%
Considerable individual variation in response can occur with cyclopentolate. While full cycloplegia has been noted in some patients after only 10 min, other cases have taken 60 min. Therefore it is considered good practice to check the amplitude of accommodation after 10 min and if no reduction in amplitude is apparent, the dose should be repeated. As a general rule 40–60 min should be allowed before retinoscopy is undertaken.

Tropicamide
For tropicamide i Gt. 1% repeated after 3 min. Retinoscopy should be performed after about 30 min. Full cycloplegia is normally brief and a third drop is sometimes necessary. Adequate cycloplegia is unlikely to be obtained in young children, where cyclopentolate is the drug of choice.

Atropine
For atropine squeeze a 1.5 cm ribbon of ointment inside the lower lid, b.i.d. for 3 days. The last instillation should be made on the evening prior to refraction, since residual ointment will make the retinoscopy reflex difficult to interpret. Before starting the cycloplegic examination check that the parent has instilled the correct number of applications in each eye. The ciliary muscle has both dependent and independent tone; the latter is small and can be discounted. Dependent tone is conditional on an intact nerve supply and this is effectively destroyed by the use of atropine, although not by other cycloplegics. An approximate guide as to how much tonus allowance to make in certain refractive errors is shown in Table 5.3.

Homatropine
For homatropine i Gt. There appears little point in using homatropine as a cycloplegic. It has a longer time course of action than cyclopentolate with greater individual variation and no more depth of cycloplegia.

Recommended cycloplegics

In very many cases cyclopentolate is the drug of choice. Although the paralysis of accommodation is not complete, a sufficient depth of cylcoplegia can be obtained by altering the dose and concentration to suit the case, as above. Only in the most difficult of cases does atropine need to be considered. When cyclopentolate or tropicamide have been used and the patient found to have hyperopia (but no esotropia or other indications for a full hyperopic prescription) it is often appropriate to give the minimum prescription necessary to alleviate symptoms. This procedure is often confused with making an 'allowance for tonus' which only applies to the use of atropine (see above). Latent hyperopes and pseudomyopic patients should

Table 5.3 Suggested tonus allowance when prescribing using a refractive error result obtained using atropine

Ret. result	Tonus allowance	Resultant
+4.50	−1.00	+3.50
+2.00	−1.00	+1.00
Plano	−1.00	−1.00
−1.00	−1.00	−2.00
−2.00	−0.50	−2.50
−3.00	0.00	−3.00
−3.50	0.00	−3.50

be prescribed the most hyperopic prescription which is commensurate with tolerable distance acuity. They may also require a near prescription which is of a higher positive power than that for distance (in the form of reading glasses or bifocals as appropriate).

Ophthalmic dyes

Fluorescein

This dye absorbs blue light but emits green, with its fluorescence rising with pH up to a maximum at 8. Fluorescein instilled into the eye is diluted by the tears and illumination with a cobalt blue light results in a green fluorescence of the dye, the brightness of which is dependent on the pH in which tissue it lies. In this way both the presence and depth of a corneal abrasion, for example, can be appraised. The pH dependency of fluorescein is an important point to remember when using it to facilitate applanation tonometry. A previously instilled topical anaesthetic (due to its lower pH) can alter the fluorescence, making the Goldmann rings more difficult to see. Indeed, fluorescein ought to be instilled at least a minute following the topical anaesthetic. The practice of wetting a Floret® (fluorescein-impregnated paper strip) with an anaesthetic is therefore to be avoided. This is especially the case when carrying out Perkins tonometry since the cobalt illumination levels are much lower than when using a slit-lamp biomicroscope with a Goldmann attachment.

Indications
  1. Foreign body detection.
  2. Corneal inspection.
  3. Contact lens fitting and aftercare.
  4. Measurement of tear film break-up time.
  5. Applanation tonometry.
  6. Lacrimal patency.

Contraindications. Instillation of regular fluorescein in an eye wearing a soft contact lens results in ingress of the dye into the lens matrix which is difficult to remove and encourages the lens to be contaminated with microbes, since the latter tend to flourish in solutions containing fluorescein. High molecular weight fluorescein (Fluorexon®) is available but its use has not become widespread since soft lenses still become contaminated, although to a lesser extent. Soft contact lens wearers should be advised that they will not be able to wear their lenses after an after-care appointment and should bring their glasses and/or the fluorescein should be irrigated away after the biomicroscopic examination.

Availability
Fluorescein sodium (P), fluorescein eye drops (generic), up to 2% w/v with 0.002% phenylmercuric acetate or nitrate.
1% and 2% Minims (Chauvin).

4% lignocaine/0.25% fluorescein Minims. See section on anaesthetics above.

Florets 1 mg/strip (Chauvin). As a paper strip (Kimura papers).

Adverse effects. None as such but see below.

Recommendations. It should be borne in mind that fluorescein is one of the most readily contaminated agents in ophthalmic practice. Species such as *Escherichia coli*, *Staphylococcus aureus*, *Candida albicans* and *Pseudomonas aeruginosa* all flourish in fluorescein solution. For this reason a Kimura paper such as a Floret is the most appropriate to use. There is no justification for using bottled fluorescein in optometric practice, particularly since none of the preservatives is fully effective in keeping fluorescein sterile.

Rose Bengal

Rose Bengal is a deep red true tissue stain which stains individual dead or devitalised cells and mucous.

Indications. Diagnosis of keratitis and kerato-conjunctivitis sicca. Can also be a useful adjunct in the diagnosis of contact lens fitting-related kerato-conjunctivitis.

Contraindications. None known.

Availability. Rose Bengal (P) 1% Minims.

Adverse effects. Mainly intense stinging on instillation.

Suggested pharmaceuticals for optometrist's drug cabinet

Note that given the choice between multi-dose droppers and unit dose containers, the former may be the less expensive option. Clearly, this is dependent on the frequency of use.

Diagnostic drugs

Benoxinate hydrochloride 0.4% – Minims (Chauvin) or Ophthaine (Squibb) 15 ml bottles.
Tropicamide hydrochloride (PoM) 0.5% and 1.0% – Minims or Mydriacyl (Alcon) 5 ml bottles.
Minims phenylephrine hydrochloride 2.5%.
Cyclopentolate (PoM) 0.5% and 1% – Minims or Mydrilate (Boehinger Ingelheim) 5 ml bottles.

Florets 1 mg/strip (Chauvin).
Minims Rose Bengal 1.0%.
Aerosol saline (Bausch and Lomb) 360 ml can.

Prophylactic/therapeutic drugs for use in the practice

See therapeutic drug section below. Given the relatively low use of these drugs, it is probably most cost effective to use the cheaper tube/bottle versions than Minims and replace them once they are used. Alternatively, if you have several practices, a box of Minims could be shared between them.

Brolene (Rhone–Poulenc Rorer) 5 g tube.
Emergency eye wash (Optrex) 500 ml bottle.
Chloramphenicol (PoM) eye ointment 1.0% (generic) 4 g tube.
Chloramphenicol (PoM) eye drops 0.5% (generic) 10 ml bottle.
Sno Pilo (Chauvin) 10 ml bottles 2.0% and 4.0%.
Viscotears (Ciba Vision) 10 g tube (gel).
Lid Care (Ciba Vision).
Otrivine-Antistin (Ciba Vision) 10 ml bottles.
Opticrom (Fisons) allergy eye drops 5 ml bottles.

Further reading

Bartlett, J.D. and Jaanus, S.D. (1995). *Clinical Ocular Pharmacology*, 3rd edn. Butterworth–Heinemann, London, UK
Doughty, M.J. (1996). *Drugs, Medications and the Eye*. Smawcastellane Information Services
The College of Optometrists Formulary (1994). Published by the College of Optometrists, 10 Knaresborough Place, London, UK

Anterior chamber angle depth estimation

Background

The most common reason for using this technique is as a safety precaution against inducing acute angle glaucoma when dilating a patient's pupils. If the angle is very narrow, then it may be better not to dilate the pupil to avoid the risk of inducing an acute closed angle glaucoma attack. It may also be used in patients who are taking systemic medication known to cause pupil dilation and possible angle closure.

Recommended procedure: van Herick angle assessment

Rationale

The superior angle is the narrowest and most likely to closure. Although the van Herick angle assessment is unable to assess the superior angle, in most cases it is sufficient to indicate whether there is a danger of angle closure. Only if the angle appears narrow using this assessment is gonioscopy required to determine whether dilation is safe.

Procedure

1. Seat the patient at the slit-lamp biomicroscope and set up the biomicroscope with magnification at the medium setting ($\sim 16\times$). Explain the procedure to the patient.
2. Narrow the beam to an optic section with the illumination system at $60°$ temporal to the microscope. Adjust the illumination system temporally to the very edge of the limbus, keeping the cornea in focus. Judge the depth of the anterior chamber by the width of the optically clear space between the cornea and the iris. Compare this width to the width of the cornea (Figure 5.9). Record the result using a ratio or van Herick's grading system described below.
3. Repeat for the nasal edge of the cornea.
4. Repeat for the other eye.

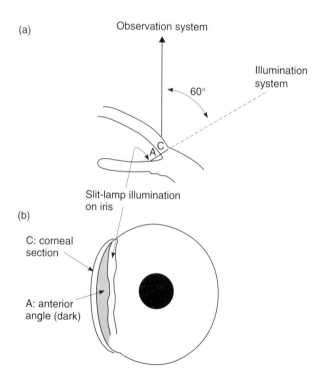

Figure 5.9 Diagrammatic representation of van Herick's technique for anterior chamber angle estimation.

Table 5.4 van Herick's anterior chamber angle grading system

van Herick grade	Cornea: anterior angle depth	Probability of angle closure
Grade 0	Closed	100%
Grade I	< 1 : 1/4	Very likely
Grade II	1 : 1/4	Possible
Grade III	1 : 1/2	Unlikely
Grade IV	1 : 1 or greater	Impossible

Recording

Record the result as a ratio with the cornea being unity and the anterior chamber width being a fraction of the corneal width, e.g. C/AC $1 : \frac{1}{4}$, $1 : 1$, $1 : 1\frac{1}{2}$. Alternatively, van Herick's grading system can be used (Table 5.4).

Interpretation

The angle should normally be grade III or grade IV. The prevalence of narrow angles of grade I and II is low at about 2%. If the angle is grade II or less, there is a risk of angle closure and the pupil should be dilated only if a gonioscopy examination indicates that it is safe to do so.

Most common errors

1. Failure to position the optical system as close to the limbus as possible.
2. Having the angle between the illumination system and the microscope less than 60°.

Acceptable alternative procedure: Angle estimation by pen light

Procedure

1. Dim the room lights and ask the patient to look straight ahead.
2. Hold a pen light at an angle of 100° temporally in the horizontal plane of the patient's right eye and rotate it around to 90°. The temporal side of the iris will illuminate.
3. Observe the nasal iris carefully and note how much of it is in shadow (Figure 5.10).
4. Repeat with the left eye.

Recording

Grade the angle according to the percentage of the nasal iris that is in shade (Table 5.5).

Interpretation

See Table 5.5.

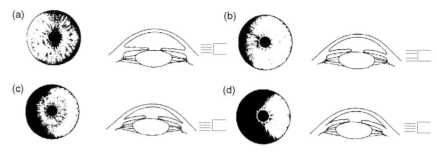

Figure 5.10 The pen light test for anterior angle estimation. The pen light illuminates various amounts of the iris depending on the size of the anterior angle. (a) grade IV; (b) grade III; (c) grade II; (d) grade I.

Table 5.5 Angle estimation by pen light grading system

Pen light grade	% Nasal iris in shadow	Probability of angle closure
Grade 0	100	100%
Grade I	75	Very likely
Grade II	50	Possible
Grade III	25	Unlikely
Grade IV	0	Impossible

Most common error

Improper pen light position.

Advantages

This procedure is useful when a biomicroscope is not available or when a van Herick assessment is impossible, e.g. patient in a wheelchair, young child.

Disadvantage

van Herick's grading system with the biomicroscope allows a more accurate evaluation of the anterior chamber angle.

Further reading

Bartlett, J.D. (1991). Slit lamp. In *Clinical Procedures in Optometry* (J.B. Eskridge, J.F. Amos and J.D. Bartlett, ed) J.B. Lippincott, Philadelphia, Pennsylvania
Townsend, J.C. (1991). Anterior chamber angle estimation. In *Clinical Procedures in Optometry* (J.B. Eskridge, J.F. Amos and J.D. Bartlett, ed) J.B. Lippincott, Philadelphia, Pennsylvania

Gonioscopy

Background

Gonioscopy is the standard procedure for examination and evaluation of the structures of the anterior chamber angle. The technique is necessary as light from the anterior chamber angle is totally internally reflected within the anterior chamber, therefore only when the corneal power is neutralised with a contact lens can the structures be visualised. Gonioscopy should be used: in all patients at risk for primary or secondary open or closed angle glaucoma, in order to identify risk factors and to differentiate the aetiology and severity of the disease; when there is risk for an intraocular foreign body; if there has been chronic or poorly controlled anterior uveitis; or when structural irregularities of the iris and anomalies of the anterior chamber are noted on biomicroscopy. Gonioscopy is contraindicated in cases of acute trauma especially in the presence of hyphaema or micro-hyphaema. Similarly, gonioscopy is not recommended following penetrative intraocular surgery, including cataract surgery.

Recommended test: Indirect, scleral lens gonioscopy

Rationale

The angle can be visualised by direct or indirect methods, although direct methods involving direct observation of the angle through a high powered contact lens (e.g. the 50 D Koeppe lens) are rarely used in clinical practice. Indirect methods use a contact lens with 1, 2, or 4 internal mirrors angled between 59° to 64° from the horizontal plane; 62° is the most common orientation. Light from the angle is reflected by the mirror through the front of the lens so that the anatomical features may be viewed at the biomicroscope. Stereopsis, magnification, and illumination methods can therefore be used to further interpret the image. Indirect gonioscopes can be further divided into scleral and corneal-type lenses. The former have a broad area of contact with the eye and are available in a range of sizes with a typical diameter of 15 mm. A viscous coupling solution must be used to fill the gap between the lens and the cornea. The most commonly used lens is the Goldmann type 3-mirror (Universal) lens (Figure 5.11). This lens has the advantage of having two other mirrors more steeply angled for evaluation of the midperipheral and peripheral retina through a dilated pupil and a central lens to evaluate the vitreous and central retina. Other variations include the Thorpe lens, which has four mirrors all angled for gonioscopy only. Scleral lenses are the most commonly used. Advantages include excellent optics, lens stabilisation even with a blepharospastic patient, and little corneal disruption when a non-preserved coupling solution is used.

All corneal-type lenses (Posner, Sussman, Zeiss) have four mirrors and are easier and quicker to use for the experienced clinician (Figure 5.11). The four mirrors enable a view of all quadrants without rotation of the lens. However, the view of the angle structures is not as distinct or stable as with the scleral lenses, so that the observation of subtleties is more difficult. Folds in Descemet's membrane can occur, due to pressure placed on such a small contact area of the cornea. Corneal abrasions can also occur especially in patients with a compromised epithelium (e.g. diabetic patients, recurrent corneal erosion problems).

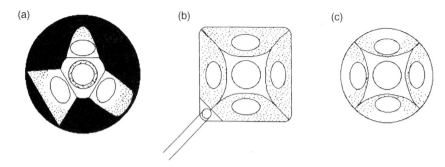

Figure 5.11 Types of indirect gonioscopes (not to scale). (a) A Goldmann type 3-mirror (scleral) lens. The thumbnail mirror is angled such that the anterior angle structures can be viewed. The lens must be rotated through 360 degrees to view all quadrants. The thumbnail-shaped mirror can also be used to view the far peripheral fundus. The rectangular-shaped mirror can be used to view the periphery, and the trapezoidal-shaped mirror the midperiphery. The central lens is used to view the posterior pole. (b) A Posner or Zeiss corneal lens with a lens handle. (c) A Sussman corneal lens. Reprinted from *Clinical Optometry Update, Opthalmic and Physiological Optics* supplement, **Vol. 16**, Prokopich and Flanagan, Gonioscopy: evaluation of the anterior chamber angle. Part I, p. S42, Copyright 1996, with kind permission from Elsevier Science Ltd, The Boulevard, Langford Lane, Kidlington, OX5 1GB, UK.

Procedure

1. Indicate to the patient what the test involves and why it needs to be performed.
2. Position the patient comfortably at the biomicroscope.
3. Align the illumination system to be co-axial with the viewing system and set the magnification to a low power (10×). Ensure the patient is aligned with the lateral canthal marker on the head rest.
4. Clean and disinfect the gonioscopy lens. Prolonged use of alcohol disinfection may damage surfaces. A preferred method is to wash with soap and water on lens removal followed by a short soak in a diluted solution of sodium hypochlorite with sterile saline rinse immediately prior to use.
5. Fill approximately two-thirds of the lens reservoir with solution, ensuring it is free of bubbles which would interfere with the mirror view. Gonioscopic, Gonak, and Goniosol are commercially available solutions which provide a clear medium and enable a good contact suction with scleral-type lenses. These solutions must be irrigated from the eye after the lens has been removed to minimise irritation and corneal stippling from the large molecular polymer and preservative. Celluvisc (carboxymethylcellulose) unpreserved artificial tear solution is the recommended alternative as it can be used from one single dose vial and need not be rinsed from the eye.
6. Anaesthetise both eyes (see section on diagnostic drugs above).
7. Hold the gonioscopy lens with the left hand when examining the right eye and vice versa using a moulded support or tissue boxes under the

elbow, or hook your little finger over the headrest of the biomicroscope.

8. Instruct the patient that you will be placing a contact lens onto his or her eye and that there will be a feeling of pressure but no pain. Ensure that the patient keeps his or her chin and forehead against the headrest. Instruct the patient to look up and, while controlling upper and lower lids, introduce the rim of the lens onto the lower lid margin.

9. Use the lens edge to pull down the lower lid further, then quickly rotate the lens upwards onto the eye.

10. Ask the patient to look straight ahead slowly.

11. If air bubbles are present, gently rock the lens. If bubbles remain a significant problem then remove the lens and re-insert.

12. Manipulate the lens through a couple of rotations to loosen the seal.

13. Hold the lens between your thumb and second finger (your first finger should be free).

14. Use a vertical parallelepiped beam ~ 2–3 mm wide.

15. Start with the inferior angle (place mirror superiorly) as it is the widest and usually has the most pigmentation to highlight structures.

16. Examine all quadrants in a systematic manner.

17. Rotate the lens by placing your first finger on the front of the lens and adjusting your finger and thumb to rotate the lens (this allows your other hand to manipulate the biomicroscope).

18. Identify the most posterior structure viewable. Use a focal line technique to identify Schwalbe's line (SL, especially in very narrow or unusual angles). Use an optic section at an oblique angle in the superiorly placed mirror. Two beams will be observed in the cornea (representing the anterior and posterior surfaces) and this will collapse into one in the angle at SL. All other structures can be identified posteriorly from the SL.

19. Use the convex iris technique to view the angle of a shallow anterior chamber or when there is a bowed iris. This involves tilting the lens into the quadrant to be examined and/or having the patient look toward the position of the mirror.

20. Angles on the nasal and temporal sides may be more easily viewed when the slit beam is on the viewing axis (i.e. horizontal).

21. To remove the lens, release suction by having the patient look toward their nose and blink (the strongest lid force is nasally) while applying pressure through the inferior lid on the temporal side to introduce air beneath the lens (a popping sound may be heard). The lens should fall forward. Repeat with more pressure temporally if your first attempt fails. Do not use a pulling force to remove the lens.

22. Rinse the superior and inferior cul-de-sacs with irrigating solution (or saline) to prevent blurred vision or discomfort if preserved coupling solution was used.

Recording

The most common reason for using gonioscopy is to determine the relative openness of the anterior chamber angle. There are several published grading systems but the suggested method is to use an anatomical recording system, i.e. the angle is graded in a descriptive way, thus eliminating the discrepancies and controversies that exist between grading systems. The anterior chamber angle is widest inferiorly, followed by the temporal, nasal, and superior quadrants. All quadrants should be inspected and graded independently. Recordings should include the most posterior structure observed, approach of the angle at the recess (in degrees) and contour of the iris. Comments should be made on the amount of pigment, presence of iris processes, angle recession, peripheral anterior synechiae, and normal and abnormal vasculature (Figure 5.12).

Common alternate grading systems include that of Shaefer which grades the angle by the estimate of the geometrical angle between the iris and angle wall at the recess (Figure 5.13). This system most closely correlates with the van Herick angle estimation method. Grades III to IV are wide open angles of 30–40°. In both the van Herick and Shaefer systems, angles designated grade II (20°) or less are considered capable of closure. Angles grade 0 are considered closed.

The Spaeth grading system uses three criteria to describe the angle. The angle is initially described in a similar way to the Shaefer system but in

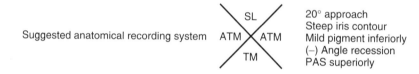

Figure 5.12 The anatomical anterior angle recording system. Recordings include the most posterior structure observed (TM is trabecular meshwork, SL is Schwalbe's line), approach of the angle at the recess (in degrees), contour of the iris, amount of pigment, presence of iris processes, angle recession, peripheral anterior synechiae (PAS), and normal and abnormal vasculature.

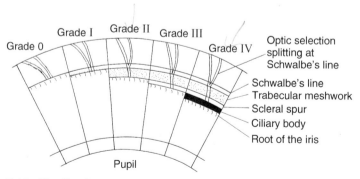

Figure 5.13 The Shaefer anterior angle grading system. (Reprinted with permission from Hrynchak, P. (1996) *Procedures in Clinical Optometry*. University of Waterloo Press, Waterloo, Canada.

degrees. The peripheral iris contour is then described as being either regular (r), steep (s), or concave (q for queer). Finally the site of iris insertion is described anatomically (see furthur reading below for further details).

In addition to grading and describing the angle, the trabecular meshwork can be graded with respect to the degree of pigmentation. The scale is somewhat arbitrary but convention describes 0 as no pigment, 1^+ as trace, 2^+ as mild, 3^+ as moderate, and 4^+ as dense.

Interpretation

The structures of the normal iridocorneal angle must be understood so that variations and abnormalities can be identified. It is useful to approach the angle evaluation from an anterior to posterior direction as all structures are not always present. The anatomical structures begin with Schwalbe's line, followed by trabecular meshwork, scleral spur, and finally the ciliary body.

Schwalbe's line. Schwalbe's line (SL) is a condensation of connective tissue that represents the termination of Descemet's membrane. It is a crucial landmark in interpreting the angle configuration but is not obvious in all eyes. It may appear as a thin, bright, white line, or a protrusion into the anterior chamber, and can have pigment associated with it. Sampaolesi's line has pigment deposited in a wavy discontinuous fashion anterior to SL and has been described in pseudoexfoliation syndrome.

Trabecular meshwork. The trabecular meshwork (TM) has a translucent appearance and is frequently dull grey or brown in appearance. The anterior portion of the trabecular meshwork (ATM) is usually less pigmented and is considered the non-filtering portion of the TM. The more posterior portion (PTM) overlies the Schlemm's canal (SC) and is more active in the drainage process. The PTM will accumulate pigment with age and in specific eye disease such as pigment dispersion and pseudoexfoliation syndromes. Pigment usually deposits most heavily in the inferior quadrant. Trauma and surgery are also causes of pigment deposition in the angle. In consequence it is advisable to grade the level of pigmentation. SC is seen through the translucent meshwork only if blood is refluxed back into it from the venous system. This will occur if pressure is applied with a large aperture gonioscope such that the pressure in the draining veins exceeds the IOP. This can also occur in ocular hypotony and other conditions such as carotid sinus fistula.

Scleral spur. The scleral spur (SS) is a white protrusion of the sclera into the anterior chamber. The trabecular meshwork attaches anteriorly and the longitudinal muscle of the ciliary body posteriorly. The SS becomes more visible when the ciliary body and trabeculum are pigmented. If the SS appears unusually wide, angle recession may be present.

Ciliary body. The visible band of ciliary body (CB) represents the longitudinal muscle and may appear black, brown, grey, or have a mottled appearance. If visible, the angle is widely open. In lightly pigmented eyes blood vessels can occasionally be observed running circumferentially in the CB. A wide CB band, with a history of trauma, may indicate angle recession. Iris processes are strands of the iris which project anteriorly onto the ciliary body or scleral spur but occasionally more anteriorly on to the trabecular meshwork. They are found in approximately one third of normal eyes.

Iris root. The iris root runs from the most posterior section of the iris and inserts onto the ciliary body. It can occasionally obscure the view of the ciliary body.

Other gonioscopic findings
Peripheral anterior synechiae (PAS) are adhesions of the iris, usually to the trabecular meshwork. Their appearance is dependent on the aetiology of the adhesion. Angle closure PAS are usually found where the angle is narrowest, whereas inflammatory PAS are often located inferiorly due to the settling of inflammatory debris. Iridocorneal endothelial (ICE) syndrome often causes severe broad-based PAS that may advance anteriorly to SL.

Neovascular growth in the angle may be preceded by rubeosis iridis at the pupillary ruff. The new angle vessels may give the trabeculum a pinkish colour before trunk vessels become visible bridging the scleral spur.
　Angle recession typically occurs after blunt trauma causing posterior displacement and tears in the ciliary body. Concurrent damage to the trabecular meshwork is the most likely cause of associated angle recession glaucoma. A cyclodialysis cleft may also be observed. These direct aqueous into the supra-choroidal space, causing hypotony.

Most common errors

1.　Misinterpreting angle structures. A narrow angle is the most difficult to interpret. Use the focal line technique to locate Schwalbe's line to prevent misinterpretation.
2.　Using too little solution in the lens, causing bubbles behind the lens which limits the view of the angle.
3.　Overfilling the lens, causing the excess solution to run over the patient's lids. Following unsuccessful attempts at lens insertion the lids can be coated in gonio-solution, thus further exasperating any subsequent attempt. Ensure that the lids are wiped and use a cotton wool bud to retract the upper lid if necessary.
4.　Inappropriately selecting the lens, e.g. a patient with a small fissure may require a smaller lens size or corneal lens type.
5.　Difficulty inserting the lens in a patient with deep-set eyes. There can be problems with lens insertion as it is difficult to grasp the upper lid. If the patient is cooperative, request that he or she look up and hold their eyes wide open, and hope that it proves unnecessary to secure the upper lid. If this is unsuccessful, attempt to secure the upper lid against the brow bone or retract with a cotton wool bud.

6. Patients with blepharospasm ejecting the lens. With these patients anaesthetise both eyes, give good patient instruction, provide a fixation target, and ensure adequate pressure of the lens on the eye. Corneal type lenses are more difficult to use in this group of patients as the lens cannot be maintained on the central cornea.

7. Using excessive pressure on the lens. Excessive pressure with a scleral type lens may cause discomfort for the patient and can often be identified by blood refluxing through Schlemm's canal, seen as a pinkish band in the posterior trabecular meshwork. Excessive pressure with a corneal type lens will indent the cornea, causing folds in Descemet's membrane. Indentation can also cause distortion of the view of the angle structures, i.e. appositional angle closure can appear to look open.

Further reading

Alward, W.L.M. (1994). *Colour Atlas of Gonioscopy*. Wolfe Medical Publications, London, UK

Kanski, J.J. and McAllister, J.A. (1989). *Glaucoma: A Colour Manual of Diagnosis and Treatment*. Butterworth–Heinemann, Oxford, UK

Prokopich, C.L. and Flanagan, J.G. (1996). Gonioscopy: evaluation of the anterior chamber angle. Part I. *Ophthal Physiol Opt*. **16**: 539–542.

Prokopich, C.L. and Flanagan, J.G. (1997). Gonioscopy: evaluation of the anterior chamber angle. Part II. *Ophthal Physiol Opt*. **17**: 59–513.

Applanation intraocular pressure measurement

Background

Tonometry is a poor screening test for glaucoma compared to nerve head and visual field assessment. However, it still provides useful additional information when used in conjunction with the other assessments. As primary open-angle glaucoma is a symptom-free treatable disease that is particularly found in patients over 40 years, routine tonometry in these patients appears to be justified. Even if routine visual field examination and nerve head appearance is being performed (so that routine tonometry is not required as a screening test for primary open-angle glaucoma), routine tonometry is useful in identifying ocular hypertensive patients who could subsequently be monitored more closely. Tonometry must be performed in any patient with glaucoma or 'at risk' of glaucoma, e.g. suspicious discs, family history of glaucoma, central visual field defect, narrow anterior angles, etc.

Recommended test: Applanation tonometer (Goldmann type)

Rationale

Applanation tonometry is the gold standard measure, and is more precise than non-contact tonometry.

Procedure

1. Discuss with the patient what test you are going to perform and why and ask about any sensitivity to the anaesthetic, for example: "I am now going to measure the pressure in your eye, which is one of the tests for glaucoma. This involves putting a drop in your eye. Have you ever reacted badly to drops before at an optometrist's or dentist's or anywhere?"

2. Make certain that the tonometer probe tip has been disinfected.

3. Insert the tonometer probe into the Goldmann tonometer and align the probe with the 0 degree line. If the corneal cylinder is greater than 5 D with-the-rule or against-the-rule, adjust the tonometer head to 43° from the flattest corneal meridian. The error is 1 mm for every 4 D of corneal cylinder, so this need be done only when the exact reading is critical to the management of the patient. This error is reduced to zero for oblique astigmatism.

4. Perform a complete biomicroscope assessment of the anterior segment prior to tonometry. Ensure there are no conditions which would contraindicate applanation tonometry, such as a serious corneal injury (see section on biomicroscopic fundus examination below).

5. Inform the patient that the drops will sting at first but that the stinging will disappear very quickly. Instil one drop of anaesthetic or anaesthetic/fluorescein solution in both of the patient's eyes (see section on diagnostic drugs above). Keep a tissue handy to dab the patient's tears subsequently.

6. Add a small amount of fluorescein to both conjuctivae. Florets can be wet with preserved saline or another drop of the anaesthetic, although the pH of the anaesthetic will reduce the fluorescence of fluorescein. Too little fluorescein and the rings cannot be seen and too much and a result cannot be obtained. It is generally easier to add further fluorescein than remove it, so give only a relatively small amount initially.

7. A check for anaesthesia using the tip of a tissue is *unnecessary* unless you have forgotten whether you instilled any drops or unsure whether sufficient drug got into the eye.

8. With the fluorescein in place, check for corneal staining prior to performing tonometry.

9. Set the tonometer scale to about 14 mmHg setting. Use low (10×) to moderate (16×) magnification, turn the illumination system to 45° to 60° to the temporal side of patient, and adjust the system to the widest beam and the high-intensity cobalt filter.

10. With the patient's chin in the chinrest and forehead against the headrest, adjust the biomicroscope to align the probe with the centre of the patient's cornea.

11. Encourage the patient to blink a few times, then to stare straight ahead.

12. Bring the probe toward the cornea. Corneal contact is signalled by either a green glow on the cornea when you are looking outside the instrument or by the appearance of two green arcs when you are looking into the left eyepiece.
13. Determine whether you have the correct amount of fluorescein by assessing the diameter of the green arcs. Their thickness should be about one-tenth the size of the diameter of the arcs (Figure 5.14). If the arcs are too thin, there is not enough fluorescein and you should add more. If the arcs are too thick, there is too much fluorescein and you should attempt to remove some.
14. Make small adjustments of the tonometer probe on the cornea until the two green arcs are of equal size above and below the horizontal line of the probe beam splitter and are centred in your view (Figure 5.14). If no pattern is observed, do not search for the pattern while in contact with the cornea. Pull the instrument away from the patient and repeat the alignment procedure.

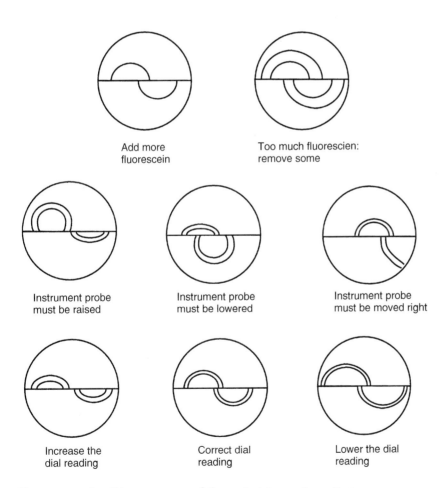

Add more fluorescein

Too much fluorescien: remove some

Instrument probe must be raised

Instrument probe must be lowered

Instrument probe must be moved right

Increase the dial reading

Correct dial reading

Lower the dial reading

Figure 5.14 Possible appearances of the contact tonometry pattern.

15. It may be necessary to hold the superior lid if the patient is apprehensive and cannot hold his or her eyes open without blinking.
16. Adjust the tonometer scale until the inner edges of the green arcs are just touching, then remove the probe from the patient's eye. If a pulsation is perceived, adjust the scale such that the pulse causes the arcs to move inward and create the correct alignment pattern.
17. Examine the cornea after taking the readings for unintentional damage and/or staining.
18. Disinfect the probe.

Recording

Record all readings (even if they are the same), that you used a Goldmann tonometer and the time of day, e.g. $_{15}T_{16}$ – Goldmann – 11.30 am.

Interpretation

The range of normal Goldmann IOPs is from 7 to 20 mmHg (mean of about 13 mmHg). Differences in IOP between the two eyes should not exceed 4 mmHg. IOPs vary diurnally, with the highest pressures in the mornings. If a suspect glaucoma patient has a normal pressure in the afternoon, ask the patient to return on a later day in the early morning, so that IOPs can be remeasured at that time. Intraocular pressure readings are only one of the group of findings considered in making diagnostic decisions. Bear in mind that low IOPs do not necessarily preclude the possibility of glaucoma and that high IOPs do not necessarily signal its presence. Visual field assessment and stereoscopic nerve head appearance must be considered.

Most common errors

1. Obtaining high IOPs because of patient apprehension. Describing the procedure to the patient in non-threatening terms often helps.
2. Pressing on the globe while holding the eyelids open.
3. Using too much or too little fluorescein.

Acceptable alternative procedure: Perkins tonometry

Perkins tonometry is similar to Goldmann except that the examiner uses a hand-held instrument.

Procedure

As with Goldmann except:

1. Adjust the chair so that the patient is slightly below eye level with the examiner.

2. Instruct the patient to look at the duochrome or other target which fixes the eyes in a slightly elevated position looking towards the instrument.
3. Rest the instrument on the patient's forehead and pivot the instrument so that the probe can make contact with the centre of the cornea.
4. Hold the patient's lids apart if needed.
5. The remainder of the procedure is the same as for Goldmann tonometry.

Advantages

1. Portable and does not require an electrical outlet, so can be used in domiciliaries, etc.
2. May be used with the patient either sitting up or lying down.
3. Some patients are less apprehensive with this technique.

Disadvantages

1. Somewhat less stable than the biomicroscope-mounted instrument.
2. Fixed low magnification for viewing the mires.
3. Does not allow for efficiently examining the cornea before and after the test as the patient is not already at the biomicroscope.

Further reading

Cockburn, D.M. (1991). Tonometry. In *Clinical Procedures in Optometry* (J.B. Eskridge, J.F. Amos and J.D. Bartlett, eds) J.B. Lippincott, Philadelphia, Pennsylvania

Non-contact intraocular pressure measurement

Background

Non-contact tonometry (NCT) has several advantages over contact tonometry, the most obvious being that it is easier to perform and can be performed by trained clinical assistants and it does not require corneal anaesthesia. A useful protocol may be to screen all patients over 40 years of age who do not show any risk factors for glaucoma using NCT measurements taken by a clinical assistant and to repeat any measurements which are high, unequal or increased from previous visits using contact tonometry. Any patient with glaucoma or any risk factors for glaucoma should have pressures measured by contact tonometry.

Recommended technique: Reichart non-contact tonometry

Rationale

The Reichart and Keeler Pulsair NCTs (described later) appear to be the most widely available NCTs in the UK at present.

Procedure

1. Explain what you are going to do and why (see section on Goldmann tonometry above).
2. Seat the patient comfortably behind the machine and ask him or her to remove any spectacles.
3. Turn the power switch to the demonstration position. Ask the patient to place a finger or hand in front of the instrument nozzle. Explain you are going to demonstrate the air puff on the patient's hand/finger, and then trigger the instrument. The demonstration also serves to clear the air passage of dust particles. Check the calibration reading after the demonstration puff. It should be 49±1 (this will vary slightly depending on the instrument that is used).
4. Ask the patient to move the forehead forward and place his or her chin in the chinrest and forehead against the rest. If proper head position has been obtained, a click should be heard. Align the patient's left canthus with the mark on the left upright support.
5. Ask the patient to close his or her eyes. With the safety lock raised, move the tonometer forward until the gun is about 1 cm from the eye. Lower the safety lock, making sure it clicks into place, and check that the tonometer stops at the correct location. Ask the patient to open his or her eyes.
6. Adjust the height of the bright red spot reflected from the sclera to mid-pupil level. Centre the objective laterally until the light disappears into the pupil. Ask the patient to report when the red dot becomes clearer at one of the four correction positions. If the patient has low or no vision in the tested eye, use the fixation light in front of the other eye.
7. Turn the instrument to the on position. Turn the eyepiece until you see the black reticule ring in sharp focus. Move the focus in and out with the joystick, until the red dot in the white circle is in focus and inside the black reticule ring (Figure 5.15). Press the button for a

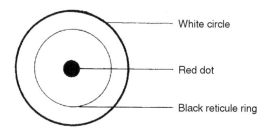

Figure 5.15 The correct pattern observed through the eyepiece when the non-contact tonometer is in correct alignment and focus.

reading when the focus and alignment are correct. If the patient is not correctly aligned the instrument will not fire.

8. If a reading of 99 is displayed, the patient blinked during the test. The override switch can be used if the patient is uncooperative and exact alignment is not possible. This should not be used unless it is necessary.

9. Repeat the reading three times for each eye.

Recording

Each of the three readings should be recorded separately. The type of reading, i.e. NCT, and the time of the reading should also be recorded, e.g. $_{15,18,17}T_{16,14,17}$ – NCT – 11.30 am.

Interpretation

As for Goldmann/Perkins tonometry. Results can be slightly higher with non-contact tonometry. Three readings are required to average the effects of the arterial pulse which varies IOP by over 4 mmHg. Occasionally, successive readings can become lower as the patient becomes less apprehensive. If high, unequal or increased results are found, the pressure should be rechecked with Goldmann/Perkins tonometry.

Most common errors

1. Not reminding the patient to keep his or her head up against the headrest. In some instruments the red dot will fail to illuminate if the head position is incorrect.

2. Not repeating the reading three times on each eye.

3. Not explaining the procedure and demonstrating it to the patient, so that he or she is unnecessarily startled.

4. Using the override switch without taking the time to position and align the patient adequately.

Acceptable alternative procedure: Pulsair

The Keeler pulsair non-contact tonometer is similar to the Reichart non-contact except that the examiner uses a hand-held instrument.

Procedure

As with Reichart except:

1. Have the patient seated comfortably in the examination chair.

2. Raise the chair so that the patient is slightly below eye level with the examiner.

3. Instruct the patient to look at a suitable target so that the patient's eyes are slightly elevated and looking towards the instrument.

4. Steady the tonometer by placing one hand on both the instrument and the patient's forehead and align the red corneal reflex with the centre of the eyepiece by direct observation.
5. Move the tonometer head to about 20 mm from the patient's cornea and directly along the visual axis. Instruct the patient to look at the red target light.
6. Look through the eyepiece and make appropriate adjustments based on the reflex seen (Figure 5.16). The tonometer will take measurements automatically once the tonometer is correctly aligned.
7. Press the reset switch and repeat the measurements three times and calculate an average (this is done automatically on the latest version of the Pulsair).
8. If the IOP exceeds 30 mmHg, switch to the 30+ position and repeat the measurement.

Advantages

1. The Pulsair has the advantage of being portable (just about). It may be used with the patient either sitting up or lying down.
2. Some patients are less apprehensive with this technique.

Disadvantage

Some Pulsairs (perhaps needing adjustment) are extremely sensitive to the correct positioning and do not take a reading for considerably lengthy periods, leaving the optometrist feeling frustrated.

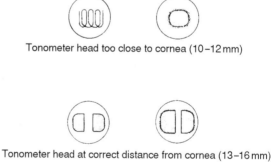

Tonometer head too close to cornea (10–12 mm)

Tonometer head at correct distance from cornea (13–16 mm)

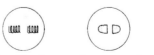

Tonometer head too far away from cornea (17–20 mm)

Figure 5.16 Appearance of the mires with the Pulsair tonometer.

Cockburn, D.M. (1991). Tonometry. In *Clinical Procedures in Optometry* (J.B. Eskridge, J.F. Amos and J.D. Bartlett, eds) J.B. Lippincott, Philadelphia, Pennsylvania

Stereoscopic fundus examination

Background

An assessment of ocular health is legally required. The traditional assessment of the fundus by direct ophthalmoscopy through a natural pupil is restricted because of the limited view of the peripheral fundus and because the picture is strictly two-dimensional. New lenses used with the slit lamp biomicroscope enable a three-dimensional view of the structures of the fundus. Variable magnification is available and depends on the auxiliary lens and biomicroscope magnification used. Many of these techniques also allow a much greater field of view of the posterior pole and fundus periphery than with direct ophthalmoscopy and are less affected by media opacity and independent of patient ametropia. Indications for fundus biomicroscopy include routine evaluation of the optic nerve head and macula. Specific indications for fundus biomicroscopy include: evaluation of the optic nerve head for cupping and elevation, neovascularisation, and other nerve head abnormalities; evaluation of the macula and for macular oedema, subretinal neovascular membranes, and other maculopathies; diabetic retinopathy; elevated or excavated fundus lesions; vitreous anomalies; abnormalities of the equatorial retina; high myopia; anterior infections or inflammations; post-surgical examination; and post-traumatic examination (also see section on diagnostic drugs (above) and Interpretation below).

Recommended test: Indirect biomicroscopic fundus examination

Rationale

Fundus biomicroscopic assessment may be accomplished optically by direct and indirect methods. The direct methods create a virtual erect image by neutralising the optical power of the eye with a high minus lens. The high minus Hruby lens (−58 D) is mounted on a retractable holder on the biomicroscope. Various contact lenses such as the Goldmann 3-mirror, QuadrAspheric™, Transequatorial™, Area Centralis™ lenses and Macula can also be used as auxiliary lenses. By far the most common method to examine the posterior pole and other areas of the retina is with indirect ophthalmoscopy with a high plus lens. Biomicroscopic fundus examination provides a high contrast, high resolution, magnified three-dimensional view of the fundus, with a wide range of magnifications available and a much larger field of view than with the direct ophthalmoscope, Hruby lens, or 3-mirror lens. This is because the pupil is eliminated as a field stop. These advantages outweigh the mild inconvenience of the aerial inverted and laterally reversed image.

Choice of indirect lens. Currently available lenses include the +78 D, +90 D, SuperField NC™ (non-contact) and SuperPupil NC™ lenses (Table 5.6). The lower powered condensing lenses offer greater magnification, so that the magnification on the biomicroscope need not be increased as much, thereby maintaining good depth of focus. The SuperField has the advantage of a high index material and low colour dispersion. It allows magnification similar to the +90 D but almost two times the field of view. The SuperField is also available with several attachments that include a yellow filter, retinal scale, lens holder, and contact and non-contact high plus and minus lens adaptors. The contact adaptors transform the SuperField into a direct lens. The high plus adaptors allow for increased field of view and are comparable to the QuadrAspheric lens (approximately 130 degrees of field). The high minus adaptors allow increased magnification for detailed posterior segment examination comparable to the Area Centralis lens. The SuperPupil NC lens has the smallest diameter aperture and is recommended for evaluation of patients with small pupils, with or without dilation. This lens is therefore useful to examine patients in whom pupillary dilation is inadvisable, or for those on miotic therapy or with posterior synechiae.

Filters. Yellow condensing lenses or yellow filters attached to clear lenses may be used to minimise glare and therefore improve patient comfort. They also minimise the short wavelengths of light that can be potentially harmful to the retinal photoreceptors following prolonged exposure. Clinicians have varied opinions on whether or not to use a yellow filter as some find the colour rendering properties of the filtered lenses unacceptable and question the necessity in a routine, quick assessment. Students first learning the technique, however, should definitely consider the filter or yellow lens to reduce the discomfort and exposure of their subjects.

Indications for other techniques. Fundus contact lenses allow examination of the fundus without the reflections that can occur with indirect lenses. This can be very useful, for example, when evaluating a macula for subtle changes such as oedema associated with diabetic maculopathy or early exudative age-related macular degeneration. These lenses may also be considered when a patient is blepharospastic, as sometimes a contact lens with a large aperture (i.e. scleral lens) can be inserted and will control

Table 5.6 A comparison of various characteristics of several fundus biomicroscopy lenses with direct ophthalmoscopy

Instrument	Image	Steropsis	Field of view	Magnification	Extent of fundus visible*
Direct ophthalmoscope	Erect	No	$\approx 5°$[†]	15×[†]	To equator
Volk 78 D	Reversed and inverted	Yes	73°[§]	14×[‡]	Beyond equator
Volk 90 D	Reversed and inverted	Yes	69°[§]	12×[‡]	Beyond equator
Volk SuperField NC	Reversed and inverted	Yes	120°[§]	11×[‡]	Beyond equator
Volk SuperPupil NC	Reversed and inverted	Yes	120°[§]	11×[‡]	Beyond equator

*Through a dilated pupil, with movement of the eye. [†]Varies with refractive error. [‡]Using 16× magnification on the slit lamp. [§]Manufacturer's claims. The slit lamp limits the field of view, therefore the instrument must be moved to observe this extent of the fundus.

the patient's lids. Magnification is variable but is often reduced; the exceptions are the Area Centralis and Macular lenses which are high magnification lenses. The procedure for the contact lens insertion varies according to whether they are scleral- or corneal-type lenses (see Gonioscopy section above).

Procedure

Note that it is possible to perform fundus biomicroscopy with undilated pupils in some patients. This ability improves with practice.

1. Discuss the procedure of pupillary dilation with the patient, e.g. "I would like to put a drop in your eyes to make your pupils larger, so that I will be able to have a better look at the back of your eye". In certain cases there will be symptoms, signs, or history which support the indication to dilate, so the specific rationale for each patient will vary.
2. Discuss the expected effects and the recovery time of the pupillary dilation on the patient's vision (see Diagnostic drugs section above). It is preferable to not have patients drive after pupillary dilation. Many patients do not have any discomfort or difficulty with their vision when their pupils are dilated; however, others seem to be significantly affected. Unless it is a necessity because of an identified risk factor, consider having the patient back on another day for pupillary dilation when someone else can drive them afterward. Ensure that all patients give informed consent to the procedure.
3. The minimum predilation procedures are as follows:

    (a) Visual acuities (with pinhole or refraction if less than expected acuity).
    (b) Pupillary assessment.
    (c) Angle assessment.
    (d) Tonometry (preferably applanation).
    (e) History of allergies or sensitivities to medications.
    (f) Extra-ocular muscle, accommodative and convergence assessment (if required).

4. Dilate the patient's pupils (see Diagnostic drugs section above).
5. Seat the patient comfortably at the biomicroscope and ask him or her to remove any spectacles. Sit at the examining side of the biomicroscope and ask the patient to look at your ear (this assumes that the patient is not monocular and that you have already set up the biomicroscope for yourself and your patient; see slit lamp biomicroscopy procedure above).
6. Place the illumination system in line with the eyepieces of the biomicroscope (zero degrees displacement). Use a slit beam of moderate width, moderate height, and low to medium intensity. Set the magnification to 10–16X, and dim or turn off the room lights.
7. Hold the condensing lens in your hand. The two other options for lens stabilization are the slit lamp-mounted holder and the lens-mounted extension ring. The lens mount is available for the +90 D only. The holder offers lens stability and leaves your hand free to hold

lids. It is also useful when doing fundus photography with the indirect lens. However, it limits the flexibility of lens manipulation that facilitates more peripheral evaluation of the various areas of the fundus. The lens-mounted extension ring is used to brace a hand-held lens against the patient's brow. This allows you to maintain a more stable lens to cornea working distance. The lens should be oriented with the bottom of the lens (determined by the lettering on the lens rim) facing the patient. Neither of these options is required for a proper assessment.

8. Look through the biomicroscope and centre and focus on the patient's pupil.

9. Hold the lens with your first finger and thumb. Use your left hand for the patient's right eye and vice versa.

10. Look outside the biomicroscope and introduce the lens into the light path, just less than 1 cm in front of the patient's eye. Make sure the light enters the pupil. Rest your other fingers on the patient's cheek and/or bridge of the nose and brow to help stability. Either rest your elbow on the biomicroscope table or hook your little finger over the forehead rest of the biomicroscope to take the strain off your arm.

11. Look again through the biomicroscope while maintaining the stability of the lens. The real aerial image is created by the lens in front of the patient so the biomicroscope joystick must be pulled straight back until the fundus comes into focus. As the slit lamp is being pulled back, the surface of the lens itself will first come into focus, then the blurred red reflex of the retina should be seen. While maintaining lens stability, continue to pull back until the fundus structures come into focus. The extent of this movement varies with the power of the condensing lens. The lower powered lenses form an image farther from the patient's face so the biomicroscope must be pulled back farther.

12. Increase the magnification and broaden the illumination as required. You can tilt the lens and/or the housing of certain biomicroscopes (e.g. Haag Streit) forward to help reduce lens reflections.

13. Systematically examine the entire posterior pole. A preferred technique is to evaluate the optic nerve head first, then follow the arcades (either inferiorly or superiorly) around the macula, to the opposite arcades and back to the nerve head, then finally scan across the light-sensitive macula.

Move the biomicroscope, the lens, or both laterally and/or vertically to obtain the desired view. Because the image is inverted and laterally reversed, what looks like the inferior part of the image is actually of the superior retina and vice versa. Therefore if the illumination system of the biomicroscope is moved down, the light will go up behind the high plus lens and illuminate the superior retina. To maintain the image, as the examiner moves the light down with the biomicroscope, the lens should be moved or tilted down slightly in order that the cone of light from the lens continues to go straight through the pupil.

14. If a lesion was noted in the periphery during binocular indirect ophthalmoscopy (BIO) examination, use fundus biomicroscopy to evaluate the lesion with greater magnification. Note the location of the lesion with BIO with respect to anterior–posterior location as well as clock position, seat the patient in the biomicroscope, have the patient look towards the lesion and introduce the lens as above.

15. Examine the posterior vitreous by pulling even farther back on the joystick and scanning for abnormalities.

16. Encourage the patient to blink normally throughout the procedure but to hold the eyes open widely between blinks. If the patient's lids are blepharospastic or ptotic, hold the upper lid with the fourth finger of the hand that is holding the lens. Make sure the patient has both eyes open. Providing a clearly visible fixation target to the eye that is not under examination significantly assists the patient in holding the eyes open. You can facilitate examination of the photophobic patient by reducing the illumination intensity, beam width and beam height, and by using a yellow filter.

Recording

Make a fundus drawing of your observations. Keep in mind that you are viewing a real, inverted aerial image, so vertical and lateral directions must be reversed.

1. *Disc.* Evaluate the health of the neuroretinal rim tissue. Record the width and height of the physiological cupping of the disc as a decimal fraction (Figure 5.17). The disc is considered one unit and the cup is therefore a fraction of that unit. This should be recorded to ±0.05 accuracy, e.g. 0.60 horizontally and 0.65 vertically. The vertical cup-to-disc ratio is of greater significance clinically. Draw the shape, size and location of the physiological cupping on a diagram of the disc. Include a horizontal cross section of the cupping showing the depth and shape, and a vertical one if necessary. In the same diagram include all anomalies/abnormalities of the disc, e.g. crescents, papilloedema, tilting, drusen, etc. Note the presence and shape of lamina cribrosa pores (circular vs elongated). Note the presence of spontaneous venous pulsation as well as the colour of the optic nerve head.

2. *Vessels.* Assess the size of the vessels after the second bifurcation from the disc. Compare the relative width of the arteries with the veins. It is important to make sure that you are assessing comparable sections of each vessel. This is usually recorded in terms of a ratio, e.g. 2/3. The arterio-venous crossings should be assessed and the presence of abnormalities such as nipping or right angle crossings should be recorded (see Figure 5.6). The course of the vessels should be recorded in terms of their tortuosity. If no abnormalities are detected, record 'No abnormalities detected' (NAD) or 'Negative', or something equivalent.

3. *Fundus.* Draw the presence of any or all abnormalities/anomalies on a fundus diagram. Do this as accurately as possible, avoiding exaggera-

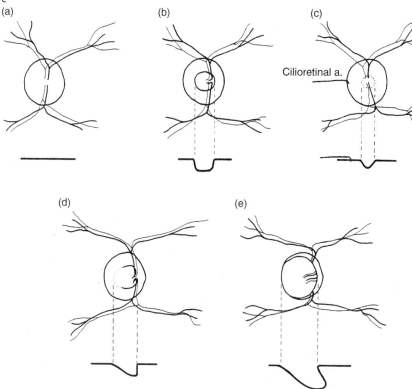

Figure 5.17 Samples of variation in the size and type of optic nerve cupping. (a) No cup. (b) 0.40 cup-to-disc ratio (C:D) in both vertical (V) and horizontal (H). Deep, with clearly demarcated edges. (c) Shallow cup with gently sloping edges and a C:D of 0.30 H + 0.25 V. (d) C : D of 0.60 H and 0.50 V, with nasal displacement of the vessels and a gentle slope temporally. (e) Advanced glaucomatous cupping with a C:D of 0.90 and a deep bean pot shape. There is no normal healthy rim of tissue temporally. (Reprinted with permission from Hrynchak, P. (1996). *Procedures in Clinical Optometry*. University of Waterloo Press, Waterloo, Canada.)

tions. Note the size, shape, location, colour and depth of the finding (abnormality/anomaly). If you can correctly identify the anomaly the diagram need only represent the anomaly and be labelled with the diagnosis and location.

The size of a lesion and its location with respect to the disc is usually specified in disc diameters (DD). For example, the lesion may be 2 DD × 1 DD wide. It may be located 4 DD at 4 o'clock from the disc. Record this on the diagram (Figure 5.18). Describe the general appearance of the fundus, e.g. tessellated, darkly pigmented, blond, etc.

4. *Macula*. Record the presence or absence of a foveal reflex. Any anomalies should be recorded as described for fundus anomalies (e.g. drusen, pigmentation changes, haemorrhages, subfoveal neovascular membranes, oedema, etc.).

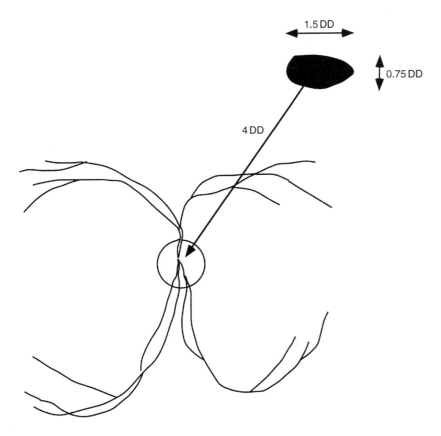

1.5 DD

0.75 DD

4 DD

Figure 5.18 Diagrammatic representation of a choroidal naevus located 4 DD at 1 o'clock from the disc. Its size is 1.5 DD by 0.75 DD.

Interpretation

There are many conditions that require stereoscopic examination to detect abnormalities that, if missed, may have a significant risk to vision. The optic nerve head is the most obvious example of a three-dimensional structure. The neuroretinal rim and cup-to-disc ratio cannot be properly evaluated without precise observation of the depression of the cup in relation to the disc structure. Often the depression of the cup extends beyond the area of pallor and this is very difficult to note without observing the disc stereoscopically. The cup-to-disc ratio with the direct ophthalmoscope is little more than an estimation using monocular cues to try to determine depth and contour. The disc should have a pink rim of tissue surrounding the physiological cupping. The physiological cup-to-disc ratio is normally less than 0.60. The different magnification with ametropia of the direct ophthalmoscope also makes it difficult to evaluate the disc size relative to the norm. This is important, as a larger disc overall is more likely to have a larger cup that is normal for the patient.

Other specific diseases that require early detection with stereoscopic assessment of the disc include raised disc margins and/or oedema from congenital pits of the nerve head, disc drusen, raised intracranial pressure (papilloedema), ischaemic optic neuropathy, malignant hypertension, diabetic papillopathy, inflammatory optic neuropathies (papillitis), papillophlebitis and optic nerve tumours.

The macula is the next most obvious example of a three-dimensional structure that should be assessed stereoscopically. Macular oedema from diabetic maculopathy, central or branch retinal vein occlusion, hypertensive retinopathy, optic pits and idiopathic central serous choroidopathy, and early subretinal neovascularisation must be detected to manage the patient appropriately. The direct ophthalmoscope cannot consistently or accurately determine the presence of oedema of the retina.

Most common errors

1. Misaligning the lens and optics. Poor stabilisation of the lens on the patient's face usually causes uncontrolled movement of the lens.
2. Holding the lens too far from the corneal apex, causing the pupil to limit the view.
3. Exaggerating the extent of the anomaly/abnormality is common with the high magnification.
4. Difficulties in deciding the position of the lesion because of the inverted and reversed image.

Further reading

Barker, F. (1991). Fundus biomicroscopy. In *Clinical Procedures in Optometry* (J.B. Eskridge, J.F. Amos and J.D. Bartlett, eds) J.B. Lippincott, Philadelphia, Pennsylvania
Cavallerano, A.A., Gutner, R.K. and Semes, L.P. (1994). Enhanced non-contact examination of the vitreous and retina. *J Am Optom Assoc*, **65**, 231–234.
Flanagan, J.G. and Prokopich, C.L. (1995). Indirect fundus biomicroscopy. *Ophthal Physiol Opt*, **15**, S38–S41.

Peripheral fundus examination

Background

An assessment of ocular health is legally required in the routine examination of all patients. The traditional assessment of the internal structures of the eye by direct ophthalmoscopy through a natural pupil is restricted both because the view is strictly two-dimensional and because the peripheral fundus cannot be examined adequately with the direct ophthalmoscope. Failure to identify peripheral fundus abnormalities such as lattice degeneration, retinal breaks, vitreoretinal traction, and acquired retinoschisis is highly probable without a binocular indirect ophthalmoscope examination through a dilated pupil.

Recommended test: Binocular indirect ophthalmoscopy (BIO) (headband or spectacle mounted unit)

Rationale

The BIO with a +20 D lens produces an aerial image of the fundus that is reversed and laterally inverted. The main advantages of BIO over direct ophthalmoscopy (see Table 5.7) include a much greater view of the peripheral retina and vitreous, a better fundus view through media opacities, and a three-dimensional image. BIO also allows a rapid assessment of the entire fundus, easier localisation and documentation of lesions, and a view independent of patient ametropia.

The BIO allows simultaneous viewing of about eight disc diameters of the fundus (or approximately 35°) whereas less than two disc diameters can be viewed with the direct ophthalmoscope (dependent on ametropia). Direct ophthalmoscopy can be used to assess the mid periphery when the pupils are dilated, by systematically asking the patient to look in various positions of gaze and viewing the various peripheral retinal areas. However, this examination is lengthy due to the small field and you are more likely to miss viewing some areas of the retina. In addition, it is very difficult to see areas beyond the equator with a direct ophthalmoscope even with a dilated pupil. Scleral indentation (see Far peripheral fundus examination section below) can be used with BIO to further evaluate very peripheral areas of the retina.

The main disadvantage of BIO is the lower magnification ($3\times$ vs. $15\times$ with direct ophthalmoscopy). For a more magnified three-dimensional view of a lesion identified with BIO, you can use a lower powered condensing lens (usually $\times14$ or $\times15$ D), but it is probably best to use fundus biomicroscopy to evaluate the lesion (see section on fundus biomicroscopy above).

Choice of condensing lens. The +20 D is recommended for routine use. The lower powered lenses allow higher magnification and may be used, for example, if the patient is bedridden or in a wheelchair such that fundus biomicroscopy is not an option. The lower powered lenses are somewhat more difficult to manipulate as they must be raised farther from the patient's eye to get an image and of course have a smaller field of view. Higher powered lenses (+28 D and +30 D) are also available. These lenses are rarely used because of their low magnification but may be chosen by the clinician who has small hands and difficulty manipulating the larger +20 D lenses or when the patient has small pupils. The +28 D lens can also be used when doing scleral indentation because of the easier lens manipulation around the scleral indentor.

Table 5.7 Comparison of binocular indirect ophthalmoscopy (BIO) with direct opthalmoscopy

Instrument	Image	Stereopsis	Field of view	Magnification	Extent of fundus
Direct ophthalmoscope	Extent	No	$\approx 5°$[‡]	$15\times$[‡]	Visible to equator[*]
BIO (50 mm, 20 D lens)	Reversed and inverted	Yes	$\approx 46°$[†]	$3\times$[†]	Entire retinal surface

[*]Through a dilated pupil, with movement of the eye. [†]Varies with condensing lens power. [‡]Varies with refractive error.

Filters. Yellow condensing lenses or yellow filters attached to clear lenses may be used to minimise glare and therefore improve patient comfort. They also minimise the short wavelengths of light that can be potentially harmful to the retinal photoreceptors following prolonged exposure. Clinicians have varied opinions on whether or not to use a yellow filter, as some find the colour rendering properties of the filtered lenses unacceptable and question the necessity in a routine, quick assessment. Students first learning the technique, however, should definitely consider the filter or yellow lens to reduce the discomfort of their subjects.

Procedure

1. Discuss the procedure of pupillary dilation with the patient, e.g. "I would like to put a drop in your eyes to make your pupils larger, so that I will be able to have a better look at the back of your eye". In certain cases there will be symptoms, signs, or history which support the indication to dilate so the specific rationale for each patient will vary.

2. Discuss the expected effects and the recovery time of the pupillary dilation on the patient's vision (see Diagnostic drugs section above). It is preferable not to have patients drive after pupillary dilation. Many patients do not have difficulty with their vision or discomfort when their pupils are dilated; however, others seem to be significantly affected by the dilation. Unless it is a necessity because of an identified risk factor, consider having the patient back on another day for pupillary dilation when someone else can drive them afterward. Make sure that all patients give informed consent to the procedure.

3. The minimum predilation procedures are as follows:

   (a) Visual acuities (with pinhole or refraction if less than expected acuity).
   (b) Pupillary assessment.
   (c) Angle assessment.
   (d) Tonometry (preferably applanation).
   (e) History of allergies or sensitivities to medications.
   (f) Extra-ocular muscle, accommodative and convergence assessment (if required).

4. Ask the patient to remove any spectacles, and explain that you are going to recline the chair as at a visit to the dentist. Adjust the chair to the reclining position, so that the patient is at approximately hip level. The supine position allows all areas to be evaluated effectively by enabling the examiner to stand opposite the areas being viewed, optimising stereopsis and the extent of viewing area. It also helps in the beginning to examine the posterior pole from behind the chair with the patient reclined so that the image does not appear reversed and inverted.

   Reclining the patient is not always possible, however, so examination with the patient seated upright can also be performed. The inferior and superior retinae are more difficult to examine with a seated patient as the examiner must be well above the patient's head to see the inferior peripheral retina, and towards the patient's lap to see the superior peripheral retina. Either way, when the eye is directed to one of the quadrants, the long axis of the patient's pupil should be lined up with the examiner's pupils to maximise stereopsis.

5. Adjust the instrument.

   (a) Adjust the headband. There are adjustments on the back and the top to allow a comfortable fit.

   (b) Plug the instrument in and turn it on. Release the lock and swing the housing unit down in front of the eyes until the eye-pieces are close to the eyes and as perpendicular to the line of sight as possible. The closer the eyepieces are to the eyes, the larger the field of view.

   (c) Adjust the interpupillary distance of the oculars. Direct the ophthalmoscope light at your thumb or at a wall at arm's length. Move each eyepiece in and out monocularly until the spot of light is exactly centred in the field of view for both eyes. Adjust the mirror vertically until it occupies the upper one-half to one-third of the field of view. This allows the illumination beam to pass above the observation beam. Not all instruments possess this adjustment.

   (d) Adjust the illumination size to the appropriate pupil size. Use a smaller illumination beam with patients whose pupils are not dilated, or have dilated poorly.

4. Hold the condensing lens with the white or silver edge of the lens casing facing the patient. This will ensure that the more steeply curved surfaces face the examiner, which minimises the reflections and optical aberrations produced by the observation light on the lens surfaces.

5. Grasp the condensing lens between the index finger and the thumb. The little (or third) finger can be used to retract the upper lid and allow for stable extension of the lens away from the patient's eye, and acts as a pivot, enabling the observer to tilt the lens in all planes merely by rocking the forearm on the tip of the finger. The other lid may be retracted with the thumb of the opposite hand. Alternatively, the little (or third) finger of the opposite hand may be employed so that this second index finger can also be used to help stabilise the lens. The lens can be moved with critical control closer or further from the eye by increasing or decreasing the extension of the little finger sta-bilising on the patient's lids. Ambidexterity should be practised and is required for scleral indentation.

6. Dim or turn off the room lights.

7. Direct the BIO light source so that it is centred on the patient's pupil. Introduce the condensing lens close to the patient's eye (about 4 cm) such that the external eye can be seen with slight magnification. Centre the pupil in the condensing lens (observe the red reflex), and align the two reflections from the lens surfaces in the middle of the pupil. Gradually pull the lens away from the patient's eye. Detail

will become progressively magnified until the red reflex from the fundus fills the entire area of the lens.

8. Keep the pupil centred in the lens at all times or the fundus view will be lost. Only slight misalignment of any part of the optical system will cause shadows, distortion, or complete loss of the view. Stabilisation of the lens with a finger from the second hand helps minimise this fluctuation. When loss of the image occurs, move the lens towards the eye again, until the pupil can be recognised and centred, and begin again.

9. Keep your arms extended with the headband unit at arm's length to the lens. By moving closer to the lens, difficulties with accommodation, convergence, loss of binocularity and, rarely, diplopia may develop. More importantly, perhaps, is that the image within the lens will be reduced in size due to the smaller spot from the narrowed cone of light entering the pupil and a smaller field of view will result.

10. If the reflections from the condensing lens block visualisation of the fundus, displace the reflections by tilting the lens slightly. Excessive tilting, however, induces astigmatism and will distort the fundus image.

11. Always examine the fundus in a systematic, predetermined order. It is also advised to examine the regions of the equatorial and peripheral fundus before the posterior pole to allow the light-sensitive patient time to adapt. Ask the patient to: "Look up and to your left...straight to the left...now down and left...", and so on until all eight meridians of the fundus have been examined. Moving clockwise in each eye is a good initial method. The novice may wish to start by examining the more recognisable posterior pole.

12. To view the different regions of the fundus, the examiner must change position and tilt the lens so that the optical system formed by the patient's pupil and fundus, the condensing lens, and the examiner's pupils remain aligned along the axis through the patient's pupil. To examine the superior fundus, have the patient look up while you direct the illuminating beam toward the superior fundus. A 'full' lens image will show approximately 8 DD of the fundus near the equator. Scan the fundus by moving the light source anteriorly (toward the ora serrata), making sure the elements of the optical system remain in alignment so that the image continues to fill the lens. Because the image is reversed and inverted, if the examiner attempts to shift the field of view the image will move in the opposite direction. It helps to remember here that only the lens view is different. For example, if the right eye is being examined and you want to shift temporally from observing the optic nerve toward the macula, the light should be directed toward the patient's temporal retina, so the examiner must move toward the patient's nasal or left side. A good rule of thumb is that your head and condensing lens should always move in the same direction as the side of the fundus picture toward which you want to see. Direct the patient gaze toward each individual quadrant and scan appropriately.

13. Now examine the posterior pole by asking the patient to look straight to the ceiling if in supine position or over the examiner's shoulder if seated upright. A single view centred on the macula may be sufficient with little scanning necessary to evaluate out past the vascular arcades.

Recording

The fundus image viewed through the condensing lens is a real image created in front of the patient and the image is inverted and reversed. Therefore, what appears to be superior fundus is actually inferior, nasal is temporal and vice versa. When viewing the peripheral fundus, the area of the image that appears closest to the examiner in the condensing lens (i.e. opposite to the direction that the patient is looking) is actually more anterior in the fundus. For example, when the patient is looking up above his or her head, the more peripheral retina will be seen at the bottom of the lens. Also, whatever appears to be located to your right within the lens is actually located to your left on the fundus.

The most useful way to record fundus findings is with a sketch accompanied by brief explanatory notes. There are two ways to document lesions in the fundus with this evaluation technique. Either way, you must recognise the quadrant that you are examining and draw the lesion to scale in the appropriate quadrant position (i.e. if the patient is looking up and to their left with the left eye, the lesion is in the superior temporal retina). Determining the appropriate anterior–posterior location in the fundus, i.e. posterior pole, midperiphery or periphery, can be facilitated by certain normal landmarks in the fundus. To draw a lesion, some examiners mentally reverse and invert the image as seen in the lens and then draw it in the correct location. Others place the examination form upside down to compensate for the reversed inverted image, and draw exactly what they see in the lens but the appropriate meridional or clock position (i.e. where the patient was looking). Both methods take some practice to master.

Scale. The diameter of the optic nerve head (disc diameter – DD) is used to indicate the size and relative distance of any lesion (see Figure 5.18).

Anatomical review. Figure 5.19 shows the landmarks on the peripheral retina. The posterior pole is bordered by the superior and inferior temporal vascular arcades and includes the macula and optic nerve head. The midperiphery extends anteriorly from the vascular arcades to the equator, which is defined by the posterior border of the vortex vein ampullae. The periphery extends anteriorly from the equator to the ora serrata.

Other landmarks include the long posterior ciliary arteries and nerves bisecting the superior and inferior hemi-fields at the 3 and 9 o'clock positions. The short posterior arteries and nerves are generally located in the vertical meridians approximately straddling the equator. The vortex vein ampullae are located at the equator and are often seen in the four oblique meridians, although many more than four may be present.

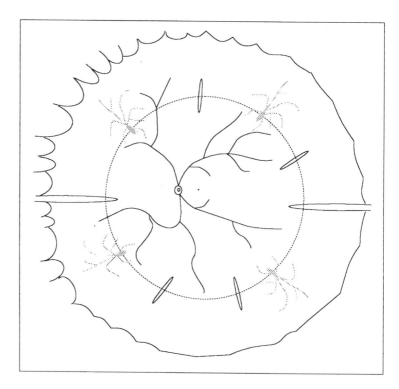

Figure 5.19 Landmarks on the peripheral retina.

Localisation. Peripheral fundus findings can be localised regarding their anterior–posterior location and meridional positions with the help of normal fundus landmarks (Figure 5.19). The equator is documented as a circle on the two dimensional fundus drawing and is located at the posterior aspect of the vortex veins. The short ciliary arteries and nerves are also located approximately at the equator in the superior and inferior fundus but are often more randomly placed. The ora serrata itself has a characteristic appearance and is drawn as a toothed structure at the termination of the choroid and retina, 4–5 DD beyond the equator. The vascular arcades outline the posterior pole. Meridional orientation is also accomplished through the use of fundus landmarks and is usually documented in clock hours. For example, the long posterior ciliary arteries and nerves delineate the superior and inferior hemispheres as they are located at the 3 and 9 o'clock positions in the periphery. These landmarks are rarely included in the fundus drawing but assist the examiner in identifying and documenting the location of the findings.

Interpretation

There are many changes that can be noted in the peripheral retina, some of which are benign and others which have quite a significant risk to vision if undetected. Benign ocular findings include peripheral cystoid degeneration, which is present in essentially all patients over the age of 8 years. Findings such as retinal breaks and detachment and choroidal melanoma are very serious and are directly related to ocular morbidity and in some cases mortality. Others such as posterior vitreous detachment, white without pressure, lattice degeneration, vitreoretinal traction tufts, commotio retinae, pars planitis and others also pose significant risk to vision and will often go undetected without a dilated examination with BIO and possibly scleral indentation.

Most common errors

1. Lack of practice. The image with the BIO relies on good technique and a stable hand. All elements of the optical system must be maintained in alignment to obtain and maintain a steady image of the fundus. The eyes of the examiner, the oculars of the instrument, the illumination source, the patient's pupil and the condensing lens must be synchronously manipulated to maintain the 'full' lens image.
2. Recording incorrectly. Understanding the inverted and reversed image as well as accurate documentation must be practiced.
3. Not reducing the intensity of the light source or using a yellow filtered lens to minimise patient blepharospasm.
4. Not adjusting the instrument properly, leading to diplopia and/or headache.

Further reading

Alexander, L.J. (1994). *Primary Care of the Posterior Segment*. Appleton and Lange, Norwalk, Connecticut

Fingeret, M., Casser, L. and Woodcombe, H.T. (1990). *Atlas of Primary Eyecare Procedures*. Appleton and Lange, Norwalk, Connecticut

Jones, W.L. and Reidy, R.W. (1985). *Atlas of the Peripheral Ocular Fundus*. Butterworth–Heinemann, Oxford, UK

Semes, L.P. (1991). Binocular indirect ophthalmoscopy. In *Clinical Procedures in Optometry* (J.B. Eskridge, J.F. Amos and J.D. Bartlett, eds) J.B. Lippincott, Philadelphia, Pennsylvania

Far peripheral fundus examination

Background

The assessment of the far peripheral fundus may be difficult in spite of a dilated pupil. Even when a sympathomimetic dilating agent is used in combination with a parasympatholytic, the ora serrata and pars plana can be limited optically by the orbital anatomy, iris, or crystalline lens. Pupils may dilate less well in older patients, diabetic patients and those with darkly pigmented irides. A far peripheral fundus evaluation is indicated: in patients with symptoms of a retinal break; when there is a fellow eye history of retinal detachment; in high myopes; in the presence of vitreous haemorrhage; and when tobacco dust (pigment) is detected in the posterior chamber.

Recommended test: Scleral indentation with headset binocular indirect ophthalmoscope

Rationale

The test is simply an extension of BIO and allows the outer layers of the eye to be brought inward behind the retinal lesion, elevating and exposing the tissues from many angles. Multiple viewing angles and manipulation of the tissue layers help to observe surface abnormalities that may otherwise go undetected or be misdiagnosed. It does not damage the retina further even when a retinal break exists. However, scleral indentation should not be attempted immediately post-operatively, or after traumatic hyphaema or following perforation of the globe. Another method of examining the far periphery stereoscopically is with a Goldmann 3-mirror (Universal) lens.

Procedure

1. Perform binocular indirect ophthalmoscopy of all quadrants (and the posterior pole) and determine the areas of the periphery requiring indentation (see section on peripheral fundus examination above). Note both the meridional location (clock position) and the position relative to the ora serrata.
2. Explain the specific reasons for scleral indentation to the patient and that there might be mild discomfort or a pressure-like feeling during the procedure.
3. Recline the patient.
4. Ask the patient to look in the opposite direction to the area to be viewed. Place the indentor tip on the fold of the lid (just beyond the tarsal plate) at the clock position on the globe where the lesion was localised with BIO. The indentor may be placed with the curve following or opposite the globe depending on patient anatomy. Direct patient fixation back toward the indentor and as the patient moves his or her eye, have the indentor follow the globe back into the orbit. The indentor should be placed approximately 7 mm posterior to the limbus to indent the ora serrata, and 6–7 mm more posteriorly to indent the equator. If the orbital anatomy is obstructing the placement of the indentor, tilt the patient's head slightly to facilitate manipulation of the instrument. For example, if the brow is prominent and in the way, tilt the head back somewhat. Maintain indentor position without pressure on the globe. Tangential pressure only is required.
5. Introduce the BIO light source. On axis indentor positioning can be determined in advance of introducing the condensing lens by noting a shadow in the red reflex in the pupil. When the lens is introduced, the optical system formed by the indented region of the fundus, the patient's pupil, the condensing lens and the examiner's pupils must be perfectly on axis to observe the indented retina. Do not apply pressure but gently roll the indentor laterally and forward and back. If the indentor is not seen, remove the lens to re-orient the view. The examiner must alter his or her orientation so that the light is aimed directly at the indentor tip. Also check the anterior to posterior positioning of the indentor. If the elevated area is seen but not in the proper position, move the indentor in the opposite direction expected (away from the centre of the lens) as the view is reversed and inverted. Another way to obtain gross orientation is to remember that when the patient is looking into an extreme position of gaze and you direct your source directly into their pupil, the equator should be

in view. To extend the final 4–5 disc diameters from the equator to the ora serrata, you must bend away from the area to be seen and direct the light up under the iris.

6. Observe all areas in question. For the more difficult temporal and nasal areas, the superior lid may be drawn downward or the inferior drawn upward with the indentor. If this is unsuccessful, the indentor may be disinfected and placed directly on the anaesthetised conjunctiva.

Recording

See Peripheral fundus examination section above. The fundus image viewed through the condensing lens is a real, inverted and reversed image. Scale is determined in disc diameters. Localisation is as for BIO. Remember that the ora serrata is located approximately 7 mm and the equator 13–14 mm posterior to the limbus.

Interpretation

There are many changes that can be noted in the peripheral retina, some of which are benign and others which have quite a significant risk to vision if undetected. Scleral indentation helps to identify such lesions. For example, retinal degenerations, breaks and detachments are much more obvious with indentation. The contrast of a break is enhanced as the edge of the torn retina appears more whitened while the hole itself appears to open and become more red. Breaks and traction may be missed without this technique.

Most common errors

1. Lack of practice. The image with the BIO relies on good technique and the stable hand of the examiner. This is even more critical when doing scleral indentation. All elements of the optical system including the indentor must be maintained in alignment to obtain and maintain a steady image of the fundus. The pupils of the examiner, the oculars of the instrument, the illumination source, the condensing lens, the patient's pupil and the indented area must be manipulated synchronously to maintain the indented lens image. Often the indentor is placed too far anteriorly, so it cannot be seen.
2. Inadequate dilation can cause the iris to obstruct the view of the far periphery.
3. Applying too much pressure to the globe or orbital rim, or placing the indentor too far anteriorly near the sensitive limbus or on the tarsal plate. This leads to patient discomfort and subsequent poor cooperation.

Further reading

Alexander, L.J. (1994). *Primary Care of the Posterior Segment*. Appleton and Lange, Norwalk, Connecticut

Fingeret, M., Casser, L. and Woodcombe, H.T. (1990). *Atlas of Primary Eyecare Procedures*. Appleton and Lange, Norwalk, Connecticut

Jones, W.L. and Reidy, R.W. (1985). *Atlas of the Peripheral Ocular Fundus*. Butterworth–Heinemann, Oxford, UK

Semes, L.P. (1991). Binocular indirect ophthalmoscopy. In *Clinical Procedures in Optometry*. (J.B. Eskridge, J.F. Amosand J.D. Bartlett, eds) J.B. Lippincott, Philadelphia, Pennsylvania

Lacrimal drainage evaluation

Background

Many patients complain of epiphora, and in some of these cases, an assessment of the lacrimal drainage system is required to determine whether the epiphora is caused by a blockage in the system. The lacrimal system consists of the puncta, canaliculi, lacrimal sac and nasolacrimal duct. The puncta are small openings ~ 0.3 mm wide, 5–6 mm from the inner canthus on the superior and inferior lids. Normally, they face the lacus lacrimalis posteriorly and can be viewed only by everting the lids slightly. The canaliculi are the ducts into which the puncta open. The vertical section extends 2 mm before turning nasally at the ampulla and extending 8 mm horizontally. The two join at the common canaliculus which opens into the lacrimal sac through a fold of mucosa called the valve of Rosenmuller. The lacrimal sac is approximately 10 mm long and sits in the lacrimal fossa. The lacrimal sac continues as the nasolacrimal duct for 12 mm further before opening via the mucosal valve of Hasner through the inferior nasal meatus into the inferior turbinate. Lacrimal drainage is an active process facilitated by the blink. As the lid closes, tears are pushed over the surface of the eye and nasally into the lacus lacrimalis. The ampullae are compressed and the horizontal canaliculi shortened by the orbicularis muscle as the puncta move medially. Simultaneously, negative pressure is created by contraction and expansion of the lacrimal sac causing the tears to move into the sac from the canaliculi. As the orbicularis relaxes and the lid opens, positive pressure is created as the sac collapses and forces the tears into the nose. The cycle repeats as the puncta move laterally and canaliculi lengthen and fill with tears.

Recommended tests: Fluorescein dye disappearance, Jones 1 and 2

Rationale

These tests are used to evaluate the patency of the nasolacrimal drainage system and the relative location of the obstruction in a patient with symptoms of tearing. The dye disappearance test allows the practitioner to observe the patient when fluorescein dye is instilled into the tear film. If the dye drains with time, then the nasolacrimal system must be functioning to some degree. If the fluorescein impregnated tears drain consistently over the patient's cheek, it is more likely that there is some degree of stenosis or blockage of the system.

The Jones I test is used like the dye disappearance test to determine if the system is patent. An attempt is made to try to collect fluorescein stained tears from the nasal cavity. The presence of dye in the nose indicates that the system is open on that side. If no dye is recovered during the Jones I test (and a repeat Jones I after dilation of the punctum), a blockage or partial blockage is likely. However, false negative results are common with the Jones I test due to poor techniques of collecting the sample in the nose.

Irrigation of the nasolacrimal system helps to determine if the system is patent by introducing saline solution into a canaliculus. If patent (the patient feels the fluid in his/her throat), the obstruction was either relieved by the irrigation, or it was only a partial obstruction. The Jones 2 test is used to determine if the blockage noted is an upper system block (in the canaliculi), or a lower system block (in the nasolacrimal duct).

Procedure

1. Take a good history. Try to assess if the tearing is due to a nasolacrimal obstruction or lid abnormality (constant tearing), or due to paradoxical reflex tearing from a dry eye or other ocular surface problem (intermittent tearing). Ask about any history of facial trauma and nasal surgery.

2. Fully inform the patient of the procedures and the reasons that the tests are to be done and obtain informed consent. Encourage the patient to blink normally and not squeeze the eyes during the procedures.

3. Have the patient blow his or her nose.

4. *Fluorescein dye disappearance test.* Instill equal amounts of fluorescein in each eye. Wait 5 min. Compare the relative heights of the tear meniscus at the inferior margin of each eye. Also note the degree of fluorescein spilling over the patient's lids. Do not allow the patient to blot the fluorescein as this might draw an excessive amount of fluorescein and tears out of the conjunctival sac. (Do not, however, allow the fluorescein to dry on the patient's face as it may temporarily stain the skin and be difficult to remove.)

5. *Jones 1 or primary dye test* (Figure 5.20)

   (a) Moisten two to four fluorescein strips with sterile saline and touch to the inferior nasal palpebral conjunctiva.

   (b) Allow the patient to blink normally for 5 min. Again, watch for fluorescein dye staining the facial skin.

(a)   (b)   (c)

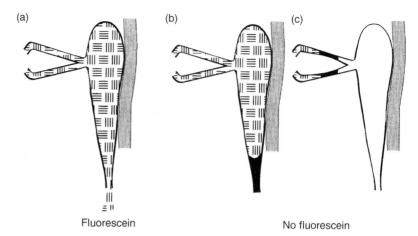

Fluorescein   No fluorescein

Figure 5.20 Jones I test. (a) Fluorescein is recovered, indicating that the system is patent. (b) and (c) The absence of fluorescein indicates a blockage or stenosis in the system and the need for dilation and irrigation, (b) shows a lower system blockage and (c) an upper system blockage.

> (c) Instruct the patient to occlude the nostril on the unaffected side (if tearing problem is unilateral) or one nostril at a time (if tearing problem is bilateral) and blow into a white tissue. Inspect the tissue for fluorescein using a Burton lamp or the cobalt blue light on the slit lamp biomicroscope.
>
> (d) If no fluorescein is present consider repeating the test or having the patient roll a sterile swab about 1 cm into the nose against the inferior turbinate for approximately 10 sec. Check the swab for fluorescein.
>
> (e) If fluorescein is recovered (Figure 5.20a) no further tests are required as the nasolacrimal system is patent. If no dye is recovered (Figure 5.20b,c), some degree of blockage of the drainage or failure of the lacrimal pump mechanism exists.
>
> (f) If no dye is recovered, dilate the punctum on the affected side (see Dilation and irrigation of the nasolacrimal system, Chapter 6) and repeat steps (a) to (e). If fluorescein is now recovered, the source of the poor drainage is likely to be stenosis of the punctum.

6. *Dilation and irrigation.* If the Jones 1 test shows no dye despite using the cotton swab and dilation of the punctum, dilation and irrigation of the nasolacrimal system should be performed (see Dilation and irrigation of the nasolacrimal system, Chapter 6).

7. Often dilation and irrigation relieve the stenosis or obstruction and the patient can be discharged and told to return if symptoms recur.

8. *Jones 2 test* (Figure 5.21). If the practitioner wishes to differentiate whether or not the pre-irrigation blockage is due to an upper or lower system blockage (Figure 5.21b and c), then a Jones 2 test should be

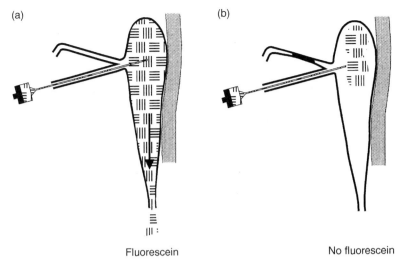

(a)   (b)

Fluorescein   No fluorescein

Figure 5.21 Jones 2 test. (a) with a lower system stenosis or stricture, fluorescein from the Jones I test will be in the naso-lacrimal duct and if the blockage is relieved, fluorescein will be seen in the effluent; (b) with an upper system stenosis or stricture little (upper or lower canaliculus blockage) or no (common canaliculus blockage) fluorescein from the Jones I test will be in the naso-lacrimal duct and essentially no fluorescein will be seen in the effluent.

performed. This can be useful information when blockages are recurrent.

(a) The Jones 2 test is performed immediately following the Jones 1 test, after fluorescein has been instilled into the eye.
(b) Incline the patient 30° and collect the effluent in a tissue or basin.
(c) Perform an irrigation of the nasolacrimal system (see Dilation and irrigation of the nasolacrimal system in Chapter 6).
(d) Inspect the effluent under blue light for the presence of fluorescein or mucopurulent discharge. See Interpretation below.

Recording

Record the results of each fluorescein dye test. For the fluorescein dye disappearance test, record if the meniscus height is equal in each eye and if dye runs down over the patient's cheek. For the Jones tests, record whether dye was noted for each test. Standard practice is to label the presence of dye as 'positive' and absence of dye as 'negative', so that a positive Jones test means that the system is OK. This is opposite to the usual convention of calling a positive test result one which indicates a problem, so it is best to just record whether dye is recovered or not in each test in order to avoid confusion. The likely site of the obstruction can be speculated based on the results of the Jones 2 test.

Interpretation

Normally, the relative heights of the tear meniscus are equal in each eye and dye can be recovered from the nose when instilled into the eye. This indicates drainage system patency.

Fluorescein dye disappearance test. If the heights are noted to be unequal, it implies that the eye with the larger meniscus may have impaired tear drainage. It is less likely that there is a unilateral poor meniscus due to dry eye or unilateral pseudoepiphora from reflex tearing from the dry eye. Most often the difference is representative of a difference in the drainage system patency between the two sides.

Jones 1 test. The test is considered positive if fluorescein is recovered. In this case no further tests are required as the nasolacrimal system is patent. The test is considered negative if no dye is recovered. This indicates a partial blockage in the system or a failure of the lacrimal pump mechanism.

Jones 2 test. No fluid flow from the nose indicates that a complete obstruction is present. If fluorescein is noted in the collected effluent, this indicates that the puncta, canaliculi and pump are normal but there is a partial obstruction in the lower system below the lacrimal sac. The obstruction was/is likely somewhere within the nasolacrimal duct.

If clear fluid exits from the system, this indicates that no dye reached the nasolacrimal sac due to blockage at the punctum or canaliculi. If regurgitation of saline occurs from the ipsivertical punctum, the blockage is likely within the canaliculus being irrigated. If regurgitation occurs from the contravertical punctum, the blockage is likely within the common canaliculus or the valve of Rosenmuller. If mucopurulent effluent is recovered, this is a sign of lacrimal canalicular (canaliculitis) or lacrimal sac (dacryocystitis) infection or inflammation. Irrigation should not be attempted during active infection or inflammation.

Most common errors

See also Dilation and irrigation of the nasolacrimal system (Chapter 6).

1. Instilling insufficient fluorescein or making inappropriate attempts to recover fluorescein for the Jones tests, which can lead to false results.
2. Not introducing the cannula quickly enough such that the punctum closes down after dilation.
3. Failing to respect the anatomy of the canaliculi with the cannula during dilation or irrigation, leading to patient discomfort.
4. Failing to use sufficient anaesthetic to achieve deep anaesthesia of the punctum in susceptible individuals prior to dilation and irrigation, leading to patient discomfort.

Fingeret, M., Casser, L. and Woodcombe, H.T. (1990). *Atlas of Primary Eyecare Procedures.* Appleton and Lange, Norwalk, Connecticut

Semes, L.P. (1991). Lacrimal system evaluation. In *Clinical Procedures in Optometry* (J.B. Eskridge, J.F. Amos and J.D. Bartlett, eds) J.B. Lippincott, Philadelphia, Pennsylvania

Contrast sensitivity

Background

Contrast sensitivity (CS) provides information about a patient's vision which is additional to that provided by visual acuity. Some patients can have normal visual acuity and reduced CS at low spatial frequencies, such as patients with optic neuritis and multiple sclerosis, Parkinson's disease, papilloedema, primary open-angle glaucoma, diabetic retinopathy and compressive lesions of the visual pathways. CS can therefore be used to help screen for visual pathway disorders and to explain symptoms of poor vision in a patient with good visual acuity. Patients with reduced visual acuity could have normal or reduced CS at low frequencies. Patients with reduced CS will have worse 'vision' than those with normal CS, despite the same acuity. When used in combination with visual acuity in this way, CS can be used to help explain symptoms of poor or deteriorating vision and to help justify referral of a cataract patient with reasonable visual acuity. Reduced CS can also explain a poor response to an optical aid by a low vision patient and suggest the need for a contrast enhancing CCTV. Binocular CS measurements, which are better than best monocular, can also suggest the desirability of a binocular low vision aid over a monocular one.

Recommended test: Pelli-Robson letter CS

Procedure

1. Illuminate the chart to between 60 and 120 cdm^{-2}. If room lighting is inadequate, ensure the additional lighting provides a uniform luminance over the chart, and avoid specular reflections from the surface.
2. Sit/stand the patient 1 m from the chart, with the middle of the chart at patient eye level.
3. Measurements should be made with the patient's optimal refraction in a trial frame. Patients can wear their own distance spectacles if the correction is within about ±1.00 D sphere or cylinder, as measurements are relatively immune to slight dioptric blur.
4. Occlude one eye.

Rationale

Pelli-Robson CS is quickly and simply measured, and provides a reliable measurement of low spatial frequency CS (0.5–2 c/degree). It can be used in conjunction with visual acuity to give an indication of the whole CS curve. It is generally not necessary to measure high spatial frequency CS as this information is provided by visual acuity measurements.

5. Ask the patient to read the lowest letters that he or she can see, and encourage the patient to guess. Once the patient states that he or she cannot see any further, indicate where the next lower contrast triplet is on the chart and ask the patient to keep looking at this point for at least 20 sec. Generally, if given sufficient time, at least one more triplet of letters will become visible in this manner.

6. Count the reading of the letter 'C' as an 'O' as a correct response to further balance the legibility of the letters.

7. Each triplet of letters has a log CS level printed next to it on the score sheet. Take the CS score of the lowest triplet in which a letter was correctly read. Subtract 0.05 log units from this value for each letter incorrectly read at and before this triplet, to calculate the final score.

Recording

Record the CS score in log units.

Interpretation

For patients between 20 and 50 years old, monocular CS should be 1.80 log units and above; for patients less than 20 years old and older than 50 years, monocular CS should be 1.65 log units and above. It is best to obtain your own norm values. If the monocular scores are equal, the binocular score should be 0.15 log units higher (binocular summation).

Most common errors

1. Not allowing the patient at least 20 sec to allow the letters to become visible when the patient is near the threshold.
2. Not pushing the patient to guess.
3. Inappropriate use of occluder (e.g. the patient can see the chart binocularly).
4. Inappropriate illumination (generally too low or not uniform).

Further reading

Elliott, D.B. (1997). Contrast sensitivity and glare testing. In *Clinical Refraction: Principles and Practice* (W.J. Benjamin and I.L. Borish, eds) W.B. Saunders, London, UK

Nadler, M.P., Miller, D. and Nadler, D.J. (1990). *Glare and Contrast Sensitivity for Clinicians*. Springer–Verlag

Disability glare

Background

Disability glare tests measure the reduction in a patient's vision due to a peripheral glare source. Light from the glare source is scattered within the patient's eye and the forward scatter produces a veiling luminance on the retina which reduces the contrast of the retinal image. In the following clinical conditions, disability glare can be a problem; the site of increase in light scatter is indicated: corneal oedema (corneal epithelium especially) and opacity, post-refractive surgery (corneal epithelium), cataract (particularly posterior subcapsular cataract), post-cataract surgery (capsular remnants) and retinitis pigmentosa and other retinal disorders leaving a large reflective area on the retina. Light scatter within the retina may also be increased in conditions such as macular oedema.

Recommended test: Pen light/ophthalmoscope with a Snellen chart

Procedure

1. Make the measurements with the patient's own distance vision spectacles or contact lenses. Ensure any spectacles are clean and not badly scratched. It is difficult to measure disability glare with a trial frame/phoropter because the reduced aperture obstructs the glare source getting into the eye.
2. Perform the test without dilating the pupils, so that the normal pupillary constriction from bright light will occur.
3. Occlude the eye not being tested.
4. Direct the pen light into the patient's eye from 30 cm and at an angle of 30° from the eye.
5. Re-measure visual acuity under these glare conditions.

Recording

Record as visual acuity with glare.

Interpretation

Most patients will show no change in visual acuity. A decrease in visual acuity of one line or less is normal. This test gives the patient's visual acuity under bright light conditions which can be reduced with media opacification: corneal scars, post-refractive surgery, cataracts, posterior capsular opacification or central vitreous floaters. A poor visual acuity in glare conditions can provide justification for early referral of patients with cataract or posterior capsular opacification who have good visual acuity in normal light conditions. Care must be taken to standardise the glare source and its angle and distance from the eye. The amount of glare light reaching the eye is inversely proportional to the square of the dis-

Rationale

For routine optometric practice, disability glare is probably best measured by re-measuring visual acuity while angling a glare source, such as a pen light or direct ophthalmoscope into the eye. The disadvantage of this technique is the lack of standardisation of the amount of glare light reaching the eye. This can be remedied using a standardised glare source such as the Mentor brightness acuity test (BAT). Unfortunately its expense is prohibitive given the small number of times disability glare needs to be measured in primary care practice. For more specialised practices, the most sensitive measure of disability glare can be obtained using a low contrast visual acuity chart or the Pelli-Robson contrast sensitivity chart with a BAT. This can be useful when assessing glare in patients with slight opacification, such as contact lens wearers and post-refractive surgery.

tance of the glare light to the eye. In addition, disability glare is also inversely proportional to the angle between the glare source and the eye.

Most common errors

1. Lack of standardisation of the glare source and its distance and angle from the eye.
2. Not directing the glare light into the eye.
3. As for visual acuity testing.

Further reading

Elliott, D.B. (1997). Contrast sensitivity and glare testing. In *Clinical Refraction: Principles and Practice* (W.J. Benjamin and I.L. Borish, eds) W.B. Saunders, London

Nadler, M.P., Miller, D. and Nadler, D.J. (1990). *Glare and Contrast Sensitivity for Clinicians*. Springer–Verlag.

6
Optometric treatment

Recording diagnoses and treatment suggestions

Background

It is important to record a summary of your diagnoses and suggestions to the patient. This is useful for several reasons:

1. It is important legally to document all your diagnoses, treatment suggestions, suggestions of referral, etc. Similarly, it provides valuable back-up when dealing with patients who return with complaints: "You never told me...", etc.
2. It ensures that you must review the case history and discuss each of the patient's symptoms.
3. It ensures that you must review the record card and deal with any significant findings.
4. In subsequent examinations of the same patient, a review of the problem–plan list provides a thorough and complete summary of the examination without having to read the whole record card.

Suggested procedure: Problem–plan list

Procedure

1. Problem-oriented record keeping constitutes a problem–plan list. Each separate problem is listed in a column and given a numerical value. The order of the problem list communicates the relative importance of the problem. For each problem, a plan or a series of actions to be taken is outlined in an adjoining column.
2. Problems are diagnosed where possible. For example, if a 12-year-old patient reported difficulty when reading the blackboard and was found to have reduced distance vision or visual acuity which was rectified using concave lenses, the problem would be diagnosed as myopia. The individual symptoms and signs that allow this diagnosis need not in themselves be listed.
3. If a patient has symptoms for which no diagnosis has been made, the symptoms should be included in the problem list. Similarly, any abnormal signs or test results for which a diagnosis is not yet possible must

Rationale

Problem-oriented record keeping using the problem–plan list appears to be the only formal procedure which has been described to document patients' problems, any diagnoses made, treatment suggestions, further investigations required, comments made to the patient, etc. The problem–plan list is part of the problem-oriented examination.

be included in the problem list. By this method any problems that are not immediately understood are highlighted and further investigation can be considered.

4. Plans can exist in three forms:

   (a) Treatment.
   (b) Further diagnostic procedures required.
   (c) Counselling. Counselling is a fundamental element in patient management. Effective counselling requires that all diagnostic and therapeutic plans be clearly stated to the patient in terminology that can be easily understood.

Recording

Table 6.1 shows two examples of problem–plan lists.

Most common errors

1. Ignoring and not listing an unexplained symptom.
2. Not providing a complete plan list for a given problem. For example, the treatment may be identified but not the counselling or vice versa.

Further reading

Amos, J.F. (ed.) (1991). The problem-solving approach to patient care. In *Diagnosis and Management in Vision Care*. Butterworth–Heinemann, Oxford, UK
Elliott, D.B. (1997). The problem-oriented examination's case history. In *The Optometric Examination: Measurements and Findings* (K. Zadnik, ed.) W.B. Saunders, London, UK

Table 6.1 Examples of problem–plan lists

No.	Problem	Plan
1	First time myope	Prescribe Rx for b/board, TV, etc. Counselled to read and play out without Rx. Coun. re. typical progression of myopia and future changes in Rx.
2	Moderate protan	Counselled re. colour vision problems and effects on career choices.
1	Hyperopia and presbyopia	Prescribe D-seg bifocals (used previously). Counselled re. typical progression of presbyopia and future changes in Rx.
2	High IOP and vertical disc cupping BE	Appointment made for fundus biomicroscope assessment and full threshold visual fields. Counselled re. reason for extra tests.

Counselling

Cause of chief complaint and other symptoms

1. At the end of the examination, you must discuss your findings, particularly those which relate to the patient's chief complaint and other secondary complaints. What is the cause (if known) of the chief complaint? Give a full explanation of the diagnoses, in terminology which is appropriate to the patient's perceived knowledge. This generally includes an explanation of what is the patient's refractive error (including astigmatism!).
2. Make sure you go back to the case history and try to explain a reason for each of the patient's symptoms.
3. It is generally best to discuss your findings in order of the patient's relative importance of the problems rather than your own opinion of the relative importance of the diagnoses.

Reassurance if no cause found

If the cause of the chief complaint or other problem is not determined, then indicate to the patient what conditions you have not detected. For example, if a patient's chief complaint is headaches and no oculo-visual reason could be found on examination, present your negative findings in a positive manner: "I do not believe that your headaches are due to a problem with your eyes or vision, Mr Smith. Your eyesight is excellent and there is no need for glasses/change in glasses; your eye muscles and focusing muscles are all working normally and are working well together and there is no sign of any eye disease from any of the tests I have performed." If the baseline case history indicated that a particular disease was a concern to the patient (perhaps due to a family history), it is particularly important to indicate that this was not detected and even to indicate how this was determined. For example, in a patient with a family history of glaucoma, it is useful to tell the patient that the tests used to detect POAG: intra-ocular pressure, nerve head appearance and visual fields (using appropriate terminology) all indicated no signs of the disease. This reassures the patient that you are knowledgeable about the disease and that appropriate tests were performed. In all such cases, always indicate to the patient that they were correct in attending for examination.

Treatment options

The patient should become involved in a discussion about possible treatment options and whether referral is necessary.

1. Explain when the patient should wear spectacles. All patients who require spectacles do not need to wear them all the time. Here are some examples:

(a) Drivers with vision of 6/9 or less should be advised to wear glasses for driving to be within legal limits. Many patients will complain of poor distance vision when driving with better VA than this (particularly when driving at night) and they should be advised to wear glasses for driving.

(b) When appropriate (e.g. no significant exophoria at near which could be helped by the myopic Rx) advise low myopes (< -2.50 DS) with insignificant astigmatism that they need not wear their Rx for near work. Myopic presbyopes will see better at near with their glasses off and may prefer to perform near vision tasks in this way.

(c) It can be a big psychological boost to a young/teenage low myope with insignificant astigmatism to be told they need not wear spectacles when playing out, etc. if they don't want to. In many cases they will not wear them anyway, and all that follows from an 'all-the-time' wearing schedule is tension between parents and child. If a part-time wearing schedule leads to too many lost and broken spectacles, then it may be appropriate to revert to all-day wear. If it leads to accommodative problems, then it is appropriate to switch to all-day wear.

(d) With some patients you need to be absolutely clear when they can wear the spectacles. If their chief complaint was distance blur when driving, it may not be enough to indicate that they should wear the glasses for driving and assume they understand that they can wear them for any other distance vision task. Indicate that the glasses could be used for TV, cinema, theatre, watching sports and when walking about outside if the patient wants to wear them for those tasks.

(e) Explain to presbyopes the various options available to them: reading glasses, half-eyes, bifocals or varifocals. It can be useful to begin this explanation while the patient still has the trial frame on their face with the corrective lenses in place, so that they can appreciate the distance blur with the near correction and vice versa. Similarly, presbyopic patients with reading glasses generally become more hyperopic (or less myopic) and presbyopic, and they can start wearing their reading glasses for TV. Patients get used to this and like it. With a new more positive near vision Rx, the TV will be totally blurred. Patients must be warned of this and may then prefer bifocals.

Possible problems with treatment

If making any change in Rx, warn the patient of possible adaptation problems. This is most important when making any cylinder changes, particularly with oblique cyls. Take note of a patient's previous reaction to Rx change.

Prognosis

Explain what is the likely prognosis of the patient's condition(s). For example:

1. Explain what symptoms should disappear with the treatment/glasses and over what time period.
2. Advise young myopes that neither wearing nor not wearing their Rx will make their eyes worse. The Rx just gives them clearer vision.
3. If appropriate (e.g. early myopes and presbyopes), explain that progression is expected, and why.

Follow-up

Finally indicate to the patient when you would like to see him or her again. If this is less than the 2 years, explain why. Always inform the patients that if they have any problems with their vision or their eyes before that time, they should make an appointment to see you.

Further reading

Blume, A.J. (1987). Reassurance therapy. In *Diagnosis and Management of Vision Care* (J.F. Amos, ed.) Butterworth–Heinemann, Oxford, UK

Prescribing spectacles

Small refractive errors

Should you prescribe a small Rx? This can be a very difficult question. Here are some points to consider:

1. If there are no symptoms, then a small Rx should not be prescribed.
2. If a patient has symptoms which are related to detailed vision tasks, you are more likely to prescribe a small Rx if the patient does a lot of detailed work and/or if the patient has a personality which is detail-oriented, precise or intense.
3. The relative certainty of responses should help your decision of whether to prescribe a small Rx. If glasses are to be of any value, the responses during subjective refraction should be very certain, appropriate and repeatable.

4. Usually small Rxs make little change to the VA and so basing decisions on how the patient likes the change that the Rx makes to his or her vision is not always helpful.
5. The effect of the Rx on binocular vision tests can be helpful. For example, if the Mallett unit shows fixation disparity with no Rx and this disappears with the Rx, then you are more likely to prescribe.
6. You can view prescribing glasses as a diagnostic tool. Often the only way to be certain whether the symptoms are due to the uncorrected Rx is to prescribe it and see if the symptoms disappear. This approach is often used in medicine. You can put this argument to the patient and ask whether he or she would like to go ahead with glasses.

Small changes in Rx

1. Even if there is no change in Rx, a patient should always be asked if he or she wants a new pair of glasses. The patient may want a change of frame or new lenses because of scratches, etc.
2. If there are no symptoms and a small Rx change and the patient wants a new frame, it may be better to stick with the old Rx unless a significant improvement in VA over the old Rx can be obtained (see What to prescribe? below).
3. Consider points made in Small refractive errors (above). If a patient has symptoms which are related to detailed vision tasks, you are more likely to prescribe a small change in Rx if the patient does a lot of detailed work and/or if the patient has a personality which is detail-oriented, precise or intense. Consider the relative certainty and repeatability of responses during the subjective refraction.

What to prescribe?

It is often assumed by students that the subjective refraction result is what the patient will get in any new glasses. This is incorrect. In many cases, the final prescription given to the patient is different from the subjective result. Here are a few points which indicate when such changes should be made. These points are generalities. They must not be used as hard and fast rules. In particular, they are not valid in paediatric prescribing and are unlikely to be valid in low vision prescribing.

Involve the patient in the decision

Using spherical lenses over the patient's spectacles or comparing spectacles to the trial frame Rx, ask the patient whether he or she likes the change in vision (or not!).

'If it isn't broken don't fix it'

Important rule for all age groups. If a patient is happy with the Rx, but would like a new frame, the only change you can make by changing the Rx (particularly cylinder power or axis) is to make the patient unhappy. (The exception is if you can make a substantial improvement in the patient's VA.) Remember point 1 of Small refractive errors (above).

Low and non-progressive myopes

'Push the plus', 'maximum plus' does not really hold true for non-progressive myopes. Remember you are refracting at 6 m (+0.17 D), not infinity. Also some low myopes tend to wear their Rx only for driving (especially at night). Here 'night myopia' is an additional problem. Therefore, for non-progressive myopes, it is often better to err on the side of overminus when prescribing, rather than overplus.

Be extremely careful of reducing a myopic Rx in older non-progressive myopes, especially if there are no symptoms.

Hyperopes

Only prescribe the full hyperopic Rx if the patient is esotropic or has esophoria (particularly convergence excess) or is presbyopic or is nearing presbyopia. Otherwise prescribe a partial Rx. All you need to do is prescribe a hyperopic Rx which is sufficient to remove any symptoms. The amount will depend upon the patient's symptoms, age, manifest and latent hyperopia, e.g. if fully manifest, then prescribe $\frac{1}{2}$ to $\frac{3}{4}$ Rx. The older the patient, the more likely you will prescribe about $\sim \frac{3}{4}-$ to full Rx. The more pronounced the symptoms, the more likely you are to prescribe more of the hyperopia.

Latent hyperopes. With a large latent component, you are likely to perform a cycloplegic refraction. Prior to cycloplegia it is important to assess the effect of extra plus over the manifest dry Rx to determine the effect of giving extra plus on distance visual acuity. This will indicate how much extra plus the patient is likely to be able to tolerate before distance blur becomes too great. A post-cycloplegic appointment may be necessary to determine the most plus that can be tolerated for distance viewing. If there is a large latent component and the manifest Rx is/appears insufficient to counter the problem, you may need to consider bifocals, etc.

Young patients

You must consider any significant heterophoria when prescribing in young patients. You may wish to slightly overplus a hyperope to overcome a convergence excess esophoria. How much extra plus may be determined using the Mallett unit and/or the AC/A ratio. In a case of a myope who reads clearly at near without glasses but gets headaches and eyestrain with near work, it may be due to a decompensated exophoria. It is often possible to get the patient to put on his or her distance vision Rx for close work and thus the exophoria is compensated. Remember that bifocals are only useful in a CE esophoria if the AC/A ratio is high.

It is easier to make big changes in Rx in younger patients. In patients over 25-years-old, be wary of making changes greater than 0.75 D.

Presbyopes

Be very wary of increasing a distance or near Rx (other than the first presbyopic add) by > 0.75 D. This is a good *general* rule for the *majority* of patients with simple increasing age-related hyperopia and/or presbyopia. Large increases in Rx in older patients tend not to be tolerated.

It is much easier to overplus than overminus a presbyope, particularly for the near Rx.

It is vital that you know what the patient wants to see with the near vision Rx(s) and what their range of good focus (and point of best focus) is. The two must overlap (see near addition).

Cylinder changes

1. Many practitioners do not prescribe 0.25 cyls, particularly when spheres are relatively large. When 0.25 cyls are prescribed, the spherical Rx is generally low and patients tend to have discriminating and precise personalities, and responses during the subjective for sphere and cylinder are precise.
2. When cylinder changes are moderate to large (greater than about 0.75 DC change, axis changes of greater than about 30, 15 or 7.5° with cylinders of < 1.00, between 1.00 and 2.00 and over 2.00 DC, respectively) generally make partial changes. Changes in power are more tolerable if the axes are not oblique. Changes in axis should never be large for large cyls. Carefully look at the change in VA made by the cylinder change, and whether the astigmatic change may be the cause of any of the patient's symptoms. If there are significant VA changes and symptoms, you would be more likely to give more of the cylinder. Allow the patient to participate in the decision if possible. It can be useful to trial frame the partial Rx you are going to prescribe.
3. Remember if you partially prescribe a change in cylinder power, an appropriate change in sphere should be made (to give the same mean sphere). It can be useful to trial frame the partial Rx you are going to prescribe.

Poor adaptation

If a patient has a record of poor adaptation to new spectacles (this should always be recorded), then make small changes subsequently.

Anisometropia

Symptoms of aniseikonia are asthenopia and headaches mainly, i.e. very few complain of spatial distortions, etc.

1. Generally, less than 1 D of anisometropia does not cause problems.
2. In young patients, the first step is to prescribe the full Rx. Young patients will adapt to surprisingly large amounts of anisometropia.
3. The best Rx for anisometropia is contact lenses. They remove any prismatic problems as the contact lens moves with the eye. They also remove problems due to aniseikonia.
4. With anisometropia ($> \sim 4$ D) and amblyopia of long-standing (age > 10 years, VA $< 6/36$), then prescribe a balance lens for the amblyopic eye, i.e. be sure that prescribing the higher ametropic Rx is going to help. Tell the patient that the good eye will not deteriorate because of strain.
5. If a patient has alternating vision (e.g. RE: -3.00DS, LE: plano, so that RE is used for near work and LE for distance) and no symptoms, then do not prescribe.
6. Presbyopes. This is most commonly found with cataract-induced myopia and astigmatism. Generally use a partial Rx of the more myopic eye (reduce by about one-third of anisometropia). Large cyls, especially oblique, may require partial Rx of power. Partial cylinder axis changes may also be made to reduce meridional aniseikonic effects.
7. If aniseikonia is still a problem and contact lenses cannot be fitted, then try:

   (a) keeping the spectacle vertex distance as small as possible by appropriate selection of frames;
   (b) reducing the thickness of the more hyperopic Rx;
   (c) changing the blank size;
   (d) changing the base curve. You may consider prescribing equal base curves in the two lenses.

8. If all else fails try size/isogonal lenses. I use this 'all else' approach because I think these lenses are thick, heavy, ugly and expensive. However, other clinicians strongly disagree with this attitude. The other approach is that these lenses should be used more as this would give anisometropes the best possible vision. This is true, but my experience is that most patients who cannot/do not want to wear contact lenses prefer a compromise Rx.

Further reading

Blume, A.J. (1987). Low-power lenses. In *Diagnosis and Management of Vision Care* (J.F. Amos, ed.) Butterworth–Heinemann, Oxford, UK

Brookman, K.E. (1996). *Refractive Management of Ametropia*. Butterworth–Heinemann, Oxford, UK

Binocular vision anomalies: a brief overview of treatment options

The precise positioning of the eyes to allow bifoveal fixation is mediated by the vergence system (tonic, accommodative, fusional and proximal) allowing single binocular vision. Normal sensory integration of the eyes occurs following correct positioning of the motor system. However, a substantial number of people cannot maintain single binocular vision due to the disruption in the balance of the vergence system, and present with a heterotropia or a heterophoria. The prevalence of strabismus has been estimated as 2–5%.

Strabismus

Strabismic patients rarely complain of visual discomfort or inefficiency except when the squint is intermittent or recently acquired. Generally the poor cosmetic appearance of the squint is of primary concern, with functional binocular vision of secondary importance provided amblyopia is absent or treated. The clinical objectives should be realistic in relation to the initial binocular status. Broadly we can consider treatment to provide either a functional or cosmetic result.

Infantile strabismus

Most clinicians consider early surgery to be advantageous when onset occurs before 6 months of age. It is important to achieve correct ocular alignment early in life as binocular development is well underway by 6 months of age. Optometrists should refer new cases for ophthalmological and orthoptic assessment.

Acquired childhood strabismus

A child who had binocular fusion in infancy but develops a manifest strabismus beyond the age of 7 years has an important backlog of fusion which will improve the prognosis. Immediate restoration of binocular vision is essential. Refractive measures should be evaluated (a full cycloplegic refraction is required), amblyopia treated and surgical realignment considered if prisms are not able to restore binocular vision. A good prognosis is predicted providing action is taken quickly. These patients can be managed by an optometrist if the condition has a significant accommodative component and cosmesis is good. However, referral to an optometric specialist in binocular vision, a university eye clinic, orthoptist or a local hospital eye department is the best course of action for those practitioners not totally familiar with the management of binocular anomalies.

Acquired adult strabismus

These develop usually from disease or injury or, more rarely, the breakdown of a childhood strabismus. If the condition is incomitant, immediate referral is required to determine the aetiology. Concomitant disorders should receive vergence training or prismatic correction. If these alternatives are unsatisfactory and a cosmetically unacceptable squint is present, referral for surgery should be considered.

Incomitant strabismus

Patients presenting with incomitant strabismus need careful examination to determine if the condition is long standing or of recent onset (see Table 2.2). A new incomitancy needs immediate referral for further examination by a neurologist and an ophthalmologist to determine the cause. The management of new incomitancy is beyond the scope of optometric practice.

An old incomitant strabismus does not need referral and can be managed by the optometrist. Patients with diplopia require help to relieve this condition. Elimination of diplopia in the primary position of gaze is usually the goal and can be achieved with the use of prisms. It is usual to neutralise any horizontal component of the deviation prior to the vertical element. If prismatic correction is not possible then the diplopia can be eliminated by the use of a chavasse glass before the paretic eye. Occlusion is not ideal but provides the patient with relief from diplopia which can often be both confusing and distressing. A final option is to consider hypnotherapy if the patient is distressed by the diplopia and is unhappy with the other options. Although this seems a radical suggestion, many patients have benefited from this approach. Diplopia is not necessarily eliminated but the patient is taught techniques to deal with the problem.

Cosmetic surgery

Approximately 15% of squints have no refractive component, providing us with very little choice in the management of the condition. If a squint is cosmetically unacceptable then referral for surgical correction is necessary. Size alone is not important but the overall cosmesis. Facial asymmetry may result in the strabismus appearing larger than it actually measures. However it must be made clear that most patients will not get a functional cure.

Binocular insufficiencies and their optometric management

These are generally minor impairments of binocular vision which result in asthenopic symptoms and/or deficient visual performance. This group of conditions is firmly in the domain of clinical optometry and provides the clinician with a range of challenges which frequently respond well to optometric management. This group includes:

1. Large or unstable heterophorias.
2. Convergence insufficiency and convergence excess.
3. Divergence insufficiency and divergence excess.
4. Accommodation insufficiency.
5. Reduced stereopsis.
6. Central suppression.

The above can all be managed optometrically using either refractive adjustment, prismatic correction, vision training exercises or a combination of all three procedures. General binocular insufficiencies respond well to treatment and have a good prognosis.

Conditions *not* classified as insufficiency are:

1. Amblyopia.
2. Anomalous retinal correspondence (ARC).
3. Nystagmus.
4. Manifest strabismus.

These conditions also respond to treatment but are more complex and require a knowledge and an interest in the subject area beyond the range of most optometrists. Referral of appropriate cases to a university eye clinic, an optometrist with a special interest in binocular anomalies, an orthoptist or the hospital eye service will serve these patients well. The optometrist should be in a position to evaluate the condition, its prognosis and make appropriate referrals.

Optometric management of binocular insufficiencies is as follows.

Refractive correction

Correcting the refractive error creates the correct balance between accommodation and convergence. Cycloplegic refraction should always be considered in young patients to determine the full extent of the underlying problem. If the refractive correction achieves binocular vision then consider prescribing the full amount.

Manipulation of AC/A using modified optical correction

1. Consider maximum plus if binocular vision is achieved, or a reading addition for excessive esophoria at near. This is a useful way to manage this condition as negative fusional reserves are difficult to exercise and improve. The increase in near power will reduce the accommodative demand and hence reduce the drive through accommodative convergence. Give sufficient lens power to establish binocular single vision and supplement this with exercises to improve fusional reserves.
2. Overcorrect myopes to control intermittent XOP/T. This procedure is limited by the patient's age and is a temporary measure. This method is unlikely to provide an absolute solution and is best employed in conjunction with exercises.
3. It is not practical to undercorrect myopes or overcorrect hyperopes as distance VA is reduced. Therefore this is not usually a viable option.

Bifocals. These are useful in non-refractive conditions with abnormal AC/A ratios.

1. Convergence excess: give extra plus at near.
2. Divergence excess: increasing minus at distance is an option only in young patients (less than 15-years-old). It should not be used in isolation but combined with exercises to increase the positive fusional amplitude.
3. Convergence insufficiency: giving extra minus at near is not a practical solution.
4. Divergence insufficiency: increasing plus at distance is not very practical as it gives blurred distance vision.

When using bifocals with children, select a large segment which should be fitted to the lower pupil margin to ensure the reading portion of the lens is used when performing near tasks. Fitting the segment too high can result in monocular diplopia. If the segment is positioned too low the patient will not be encouraged to use this portion of the lens and the binocular anomaly will remain.

To calculate a tentative add lens power, a theoretical estimate can be made by measuring the AC/A ratio using the heterophoria method. In a case of convergence excess:

$$\text{Dist. } 2^{\Delta} \text{ esophoria}$$

$$\text{Near } 14^{\Delta} \text{ esophoria}$$

$$\text{PD } 60\,\text{mm}$$
$$\text{AC/A} = 6 + \frac{(14 - 2)}{3}$$
$$\text{AC/A} = 10^{\Delta}/\text{D}$$

$$\text{Add lens for near} = -1.25\,\text{D}$$

This provides a starting point for evaluation of binocular status. Measure heterophoria using the cover test and fusional recovery rate.

Fixation disparity The amount of overcorrection or add can be estimated form the size of additional spherical lens required to neutralise the appropriate fixation disparity.

Prismatic correction

Prismatic correction is mainly used in the treatment of unstable heterophoria and to relieve diplopia in the primary position of an old and well investigated incomitant squint (see above). When correcting heterophoria be aware of prism adaptation. Clinically, there are two main criteria in the prescribing of prism: Sheard's criterion and prism neutralisation of fixation disparity.

Sheard's criterion This states that: the compensating vergence should be at least twice the heterophoria amplitude. This can be calculated by measuring the heterophoria and the compensating vergence.

$$\text{Sheard prism} = \tfrac{2}{3}(\text{phoria}) - \tfrac{1}{3}(\text{compensating vergence})$$

e.g. a patient with 10^Δ exophoria at near and a compensating vergence of 11 base-out would require the following prism for correction:

$$\text{Sheard prism} = \frac{(2\times10)-11}{3}$$

$$\text{Prism} = 3^\Delta \text{ IN}$$

Fixation disparity. Only prescribe prism to patients with symptoms. Many patients have a fixation disparity but have no visual difficulty. Remember that the amount of prism to neutralise the disparity is not always related to the angular subtense of the error, as adaptation plays a key role in the stability of the oculomotor system. The Mallett unit remains the most popular test used within the UK and provides a good starting point in the selection of prism.

Vision training

Vision training is preferred to surgery or optical correction as it provides the best possibility of a functional cure. The aim is to give stable, comfortable, functional binocular vision. This form of therapy is often used in conjunction with the above treatments. Techniques used in vision training include the following.

Physiological diplopia. This technique ensures that check markers are used to control eye position, as they help to break down suppression. If binocular vision is present at one fixation distance then in principle it should be possible to achieve binocularity at all distances. This procedure is preferred to simple pen-to-nose exercises which can allow the patient to suppress the image of a deviating eye.

Near-to-far tracking. Pen-to-nose exercise is the usual variant of this test as it is simple to perform and easily understood by patients. Care is required as fusion is not always achieved but no diplopia is reported due to a well developed suppression mechanism.

Step-vergence. Introduce a loose prism before the eyes while the patient fixates a target. Disparity is introduced and the vergence system is stimulated to retain fusion. The prism is removed once fusion is established. A series of repetitions is performed to strengthen fusion.

Sliding vergence. A target is fixated through a variable prism stereoscope or a Risley prism and the amount of prism is increased to blur/break/recovery. Repeated trials can improve the fusional amplitude.

Near-to-far jumps. Exercise accommodation and vergence together. The patient alternates fixation between targets of different distances and must maintain clear single vision at all fixation distances.

Training accommodation.

Accommodation insufficiency is often reported in puberty and is often associated with convergence insufficiency.

Symptoms. Discomfort, intermittent blur, headaches, blur at distance after reading and vice-versa.

Signs. Low amplitude of accommodation, which gets worse on repeated measures. Patients report target alternately blurred and clear when performing task. Reduced accommodation facility.

Norms for accommodation facility (fixation distance 33 cm):
Adult (± 1.50 D) 20 cycles in 60–65 sec is normal; > 90 sec is abnormal.
Child (± 2.00 D) 10 cycles in 50–55 sec is normal; > 75 sec is abnormal.

A cycloplegic refraction should be performed to rule out latent hyperopia and pseudomyopia.

Treatment. Reading spectacles or bifocals with associated base-in prism to relieve the stress on the vergence system. Alternatively, the following vision training has been shown to be successful:

1. Push-up or physiological diplopia.
2 Jump focus.
3. Monocular and binocular accommodative rock.

Overview of treatment

It is important to conduct a full examination of the patient to arrive at the correct diagnosis and hopefully identify the cause of the condition. The importance of treatment should be discussed with the patient or their guardian and the consequences of not following an agreed course of action considered. It is important to consider the prognosis of the condition and determine a plan of management within a realistic time frame. Patients will be more likely to comply if they understand fully the implications of the management strategy and the time scale. Alternative management methods should be carefully considered to suit the patient. Older patients may not be happy to follow exercises with a long term goal of relieving symptoms but require an immediate solution to allow continuation with work or hobbies. It is important to realise that the course of action is not determined by optometric considerations alone.

Further reading

Ciuffreda, K.J., Levi, D.M. and Selenow, A. (1991). *Amblyopia: Basic and Clinical Aspects.* Butterworth-Heinemann, Oxford, UK

Stidwell, D. (1990). *Orthoptic Assessment and Management* Blackwell Scientific Publications, Oxford, UK

van Noorden, G.K. (1980). *Binocular Vision and Ocular Motility; Theory and Management of Strabismus.* C.V. Mosby, St. Louis, Missouri

Prophylactic and therapeutic drugs

Notes

See Diagnostic drugs section in Chapter 5. In addition, it should be noted that:

1. Availability of drugs in the following text has been restricted to those which the optometrist can legally obtain/supply/use and which are in more common clinical use.
2. Drugs such as sodium sulphacetamide and oxyphenbutazone fall into the category of drugs which have ceased to be commercially available.
3. Some prophylactic/therapeutic drugs, such as chloramphenicol drops, need to be refrigerated.

Background

See Diagnostic drugs section in Chapter 5 for an outline of the legislation which serves to describe the circumstances in which optometrists may use drugs, and to categorise medicines into the following three product groups:

1. General sales list (GSL).
2. Pharmacy medicines (P).
3. Prescription only medicines (PoM).

Rationale

The use of drugs can be categorised as those used in prophylaxis or those used in the treatment of established disease. In either of these instances it is essential that the clinician balances the risk of treatment, with due regard to any possible adverse effects, for example, against the risk of non-intervention. The optometrist should also bear in mind the legal obligations, as outlined at the beginning of the section on diagnostic drugs in Chapter 5.

Basically, the supply of drugs by optometrists must be in line with their professional practice and the situation be an emergency. These terms are difficult to define and the legislation leaves the onus somewhat on the optometrist to decide whether a patient should be treated. Both prophylactic and emergency use or supply of drugs clearly fall within the optometrist's remit and each case must therefore be considered on its own merits with due regard to the availability of medical care.

Consider the following cases, which illustrate some likely scenarios:

Case 1. A patient with a deep corneal laceration attends an optometrist who has a practice 200 metres from a hospital eye department. The obvious action here would be to refer the patient immediately without initiating treatment. If, on the other hand, the practice was an 8 hour journey from specialist care, then this would be considered an emergency and the appropriate treatment should be given immediately.

Case 2. On a late summer afternoon a young patient attends an optometrist who has a rural practice. The area is serviced on a weekly basis by a general practitioner, who is not available for several days. The optometrist makes a diagnosis of acute seasonal conjunctivitis. Although the condition is acute, its management does not warrant emergency hospital care and can be managed legitimately by the optometrist. Of course, a report must be sent to the GP. If the diagnosis was vernal conjunctivitis, however, because of its sight-threatening nature and the need for steroids (which optometrists are currently unable to use or supply), the patient would need referral for emergency care.

In summary, the decision to treat a patient must be made on:

1. The nature of the condition itself.
2. Accessibility of appropriate medical care.
3. Legal availability of suitable drugs to treat the condition.

Prophylactic drugs

Antiseptic agents

Indications. To prevent secondary infection in minor corneal abrasions. In this case, best practice probably dictates that the optometrist should supply the pharmaceutical.

Contraindications. Known sensitivity to dibromopropamidine isethionate or preservatives.

Available antiseptic agents
Propamidine isethionate (P) 0.1% – Brolene (Rhone–Poulenc Rorer) 10 ml bottles, Golden Eye ointment, 10 ml bottles (Typharm).
Dibromopropamidine Isethionate (P) 0.15% ointments – Brolene 5 g tube, Golden Eye ointment 5 g tube.

Adverse effects. Hypersensitivity can occur, in which case discontinue.

Suggested dosage regimen. Ung 0.15% b.i.d. or p.r.n., drops p.r.n.

Conjunctival decongestants

Indications. To render an irritated red eye white after contact lens procedures, contact tonometry, gonioscopy, or ultrasonography.

Contraindications. Known sensitivity to phenylephrine or preservatives. Cardiovascular reactions (due to the sympathomimetic effects) are unlikely with a low dose in normal patients but older people, especially those with a history of cardiovascular problems, should certainly avoid their regular use.

Available conjunctival decongestants
Phenylephrine hydrochloride (P) 0.12% – Isopto frin (Alcon), 10 ml bottle.

Adverse effects. May induce slight mydriasis and therefore an associated minimal risk of closed angle glaucoma. Occasionally, rebound hyperaemia occurs with prolonged use. It should be noted that the above and their related products (such as those containing naphazoline and antazoline) are meant for occasional use and under no circumstances should be used purely for cosmesis on a regular basis. If used in this way as a so-called 'eye whitener', rebound hyperaemia is more likely, as are the chances of an adverse cardio-vascular effect.

Suggested dosage regimen. i Gt. p.r.n.

Ocular lubricants

Indications. For emergency lubrication after trauma, which may include uncomplicated superficial corneal abrasions whatever the cause.

Contraindications. True lubricants should not be used in occasions where there is active allergic/chlamydial keratoconjunctivitis. The goal in these cases is to manage the underlying cause rather than masking the symptoms by providing lubrication.

Available lubricants. There are many agents currently being marketed for ocular lubrication. The following are perhaps the better products to consider following trauma, since they contain true lubricants such as petrolatum, mineral oils, lanolin and yellow soft paraffin. Some examples are:

Lacri-Lube ointment (P) (Allergan) 3.5 g and 5 g tubes.
Lubrifilm ointment (P) (Cusi) 4 g tubes.

Eyewashes and irrigating solutions

Indications
1. To remove allergens or remnants of solutions used in ophthalmic procedures such as tonometry or gonioscopy.

2. Emergency irrigation after chemical splash.

Contraindications. Sensitivity to any preservatives in the formulation.

Available eyewashes. For normal clinical use a buffered sterile saline solution is quite adequate such as:

Sodium chloride 0.9% w/v (GSL) – Sterac (Galen) 150 ml bottle, Bausch and Lomb aerosol saline 360 ml can.
Minims (P) (Chauvin) unit dose.

Note that aerosol saline should not be squirted directly into the eye but should be put into a clean vessel suitable for irrigating purposes prior to instillation.

Available irrigating solutions. Although copious amounts of tap water can be used in an emergency the availability of a large volume of a sterile eyewash in a container incorporating an eye bath/cup is preferable, e.g.:

Sodium chloride 0.9% w/v (GSL) – Emergency eye wash (Optrex) 500 ml bottle.

Artificial tears

These preparations, as opposed to ocular lubricants, are generally formulated to be similar to natural tears. They therefore tend to contain polymers, some salts to mimic the properties of tears and an aqueous vehicle. Most patients will require only occasional relief from the burning–itching sensation of dry eye which is often associated with dry atmospheres and possibly longer periods of VDU use. These symptoms can be relieved with artificial tears, which are normally pharmacy medicines. The optometrist is probably in the best position to make the diagnosis and give useful advice on the value of these products. A report of the diagnosis and suggested treatment should be made to the GP. The dose should be q. 4 h initially to determine efficacy and p.r.n. thereafter. There are many 'artificial tear' products and those listed below are only a small selection.

Keratoconjunctivitis sicca is probably best treated ophthalmologically since there may well be underlying systemic disease which will involve further investigation.

Simple artificial tears
Hypromellose (P) 0.5% (generic), Isopto plain (Alcon) 10 ml bottles and others.
Polyvinyl alcohol (P) 1% – Hypotears (Iolab) 10 ml bottles and others.
Hydroxymethylcellulose (P) 0.44% with 0.35% sodium chloride – Minims (Chauvin).

Artificial tears with extra polymers
Polyacrylic acid (P) 0.2% – Viscotears (Ciba Vision) 10 g tube (gel).

Lid scrubs

Lid scrubbing is a useful adjunct to the treatment of acute and chronic infections of the eyelids. Many GPs are unaware of the importance of lid hygiene in supplementing topical antibiotic ointment and not infrequently optometrists can suggest lid scrubbing to good effect. A report of any diagnosis and suggested treatment should be made to the GP. Although a solution of baby shampoo diluted 50:50 with warm water can be used for lid margin hygiene, commercially available lid scrub products (normally pre-moistened gauze or cotton pads) such as Lid Care (Ciba Vision) cause potentially less stinging and toxicity. They are efficient in removing oils, debris and desquamated skin associated with lid infection.

Therapeutic drugs

Indications for therapeutics

1. Bacterial infections, in what may be considered to be an emergency situation or greater possibility of secondary infection caused by deeper and more serious corneal abrasions.
2. Seasonal and perennial allergies caused by hay fever or dust mite, for example.
3. Emergency treatment of closed angle glaucoma (or to reverse mydriasis).
4. Emergency treatment of acute anterior uveitis/cyclitis.

Anti-infectives

Contraindications. Known sensitivity to chloramphenicol or preservatives. Contact lens wear during treatment.

Available anti-infectives
Chloramphenicol (PoM) eye drops 0.5% (generic) 10 ml bottle, Minims, Sno Phenicol (Chauvin) 10 ml bottle, Chlormycetin Redidrops (Parke–Davis) 5 and 10 ml bottles.
Chloramphenicol (PoM) eye ointment 1.0% (generic) 4 g tube, Chlormycetin (Parke–Davis) 4 g tube.
Framycetin (PoM use only) eye drops 0.5% – Soframycin (Roussel).
Framycetin (PoM use only) eye ointment 0.5% – Soframycin.

Adverse effects. Rarely, cases of aplastic anaemia have been reported following very prolonged ocular use of chloramphenicol.

Suggested dosage regimen. Antibiotics must be used for at least 5 days in order to circumvent bacterial resistance; Gt. 0.5% b.i.d. or q.i.d. ung 1% b.i.d. Ointment is best used just before bedtime (since ointment tends to blur vision during waking hours), with drops being reserved for daytime use.

Framycetin cannot be supplied to a patient. This legal classification means that without asking the patient to attend for appointments twice a day, it is impossible to comply with standard practice of antibiotic use in relation to completing treatment. If only for this reason, chloramphenicol should be considered the anti-infective agent of choice.

Anti-histamines

Mild ocular manifestations of hayfever can be treated by antazoline. This is a useful antihistamine drug (H_1 blocker) used in combination with a vasoconstrictor, which helps to improve the comfort and appearance of a mildly irritated allergic eye. More severe cases of allergy usually need to be dealt with by adding systemic anti-histamines, many of which are now pharmacy medications and can easily be recommended to patients (see below).

Contraindications. Known sensitivity to antazoline, xylometazoline, naphazoline or preservatives. Contact lens wear during treatment.

Available anti-histamines
Antazoline (P) 0.5% eye drops (marketed in combination with the sympathomimetic vasoconstrictor xylometazoline as Otrovine–Antistin (Ciba) 10 ml bottles, and also as Vascon-A (Iolab) 10 ml bottles, in combination with another sympathomimetic vasoconstrictor – naphazoline.

Adverse effects. Occasionally, transient stinging.

Suggested dosage regimen. Ad Gt. b.i.d. or t.i.d. Lowest dose in children.

Mast cell stabilisers

Mast cell stabilisers are an effective prophylactic treatment for seasonal conjunctivitis. It should be noted that because mast cell stabilisers have no effect on inflammatory mediators which have already been released, the beneficial effects may take several weeks to become apparent. During this time it is essential that the patient uses the product continually on a q. 4 h or q. 6 h basis.

Indications. For the prophylactic treatment of seasonal conjunctivitis and other ocular allergies. A report of any diagnosis and suggested treatment should be made to the GP.

Contraindications. None cited in the literature but sodium cromoglycate is known to be less satisfactory in chronic allergic conditions.

Available mast cell stabilisers
Sodium cromoglycate (P) – Opticrom allergy eye drops (Fisons) Hay-Crom (Baker Norton) and others, all in 5 or 10 ml bottles.

The legal classification of this drug can be somewhat confusing. It is available in 5 and 10 ml bottles as allergy or hay fever eye drops in 2% solution as a pharmacy medicine. Therefore an optometrist can obtain this version of sodium cromoglycate and supply it to a patient. When intended for chronic (rather than seasonal) purposes, the preparation would be in a 13.5 ml bottle in either 2% or 4% ointment and labelled as a prescription only medicine and thus cannot be obtained, used or supplied by an optometrist.

It may be that purely topical treatment is inadequate to control an acute allergic reaction. In these cases it may be within the optometrist's remit to recommend the appropriate systemic pharmacy medicines or those from the general sales list (GSL). If this is the case, then the newer anti-histamines, which do not cross the blood–brain barrier, such as terfenadine as opposed to the older antihistamines like chlorpheniramine are the best choice, particularly for those patients who drive or operate machinery, since they are said to cause less drowsiness.

Vernal conditions and contact lens related conjunctivitis respond less well to sodium cromoglycate and, although useful, other drugs such as steroids (unavailable to optometrists) are the treatment of first choice.

Ocular anti-hypertensives (miotics)

Indications

1. For the reversal of mydriasis or the emergency treatment of closed angle glaucoma. The routine reversal of mydriasis caused by antimuscarinic agents is rarely needed since the time scale of action of tropicamide (especially the 0.5% concentration) is short enough to prevent great patient inconvenience. In certain situations, perhaps where a patient is particularly photophobic or wishes to drive, reversal may be considered by using a cholinergic agonist. Whatever the drug used for non-emergency reversal, one drop of the lowest concentration of the miotics below is adequate.
2. For the emergency treatment of acute closed angle glaucoma. These cases can occur either as a result of pharmacological mydriasis or spontaneously, are an important optometric emergency, and it is essential that such cases are immediately diagnosed.

Signs and symptoms of angle closure include:

(a) Moderate to intense ocular pain.
(b) Blurring or haziness of vision.
(c) Markedly increased intraocular pressure.
(d) General conjunctival hyperaemia and injection.
(e) Mid-dilated pupil.
(f) Haziness of the corneal stroma.
(g) A closed anterior chamber angle as seen by gonioscopy.

Contraindications

1. Known sensitivity to any of the drugs below.

2. Use of cholinergic agonists in high myopes or those with a personal history or family history of retinal detachment should be avoided because the stress on the retina caused by any ciliary spasm can tear susceptible retinas.
3. Mydriasis caused by phenylephrine should not be reversed with cholinergic agonists since this results in both dilator and sphincter muscles being stimulated, thereby pulling the iris in opposite directions.

Available ocular anti-hypertensive/miotic agents
Carbachol (PoM) 3%– Isopto Carbachol (Alcon). 10 ml bottles.
Physostigmine sulphate (PoM) (Eserine) 0.25% and 0.5% (generic) 10 ml bottles.
Pilocarpine hydrochloride/nitrate (PoM) 0.5%, 1%, 2%, 3% and 4% (generic) 10 ml bottles, 1%, 2% and 4% Minims and Sno Pilo (Chauvin) 10 ml bottles, 1%, 2%, 3% and 4% Isopto carpine (Alcon) 10 ml bottles.

Suggested action/dosage regimen. Should the above signs and symptoms occur, it is absolutely essential that the depth of the anterior chamber angle be checked and tonometry performed to confirm the diagnosis of angle closure. You should respond in one of the following ways:

1. Arrange a direct ophthalmological referral for immediate emergency care

or

2. Initiate emergency optometric treatment for acute angle closure followed by referral to the patient's general practitioner when the IOP has reduced to an acceptable level. An early ophthalmological opinion should be recommended since such patients are clearly in danger of future closed angle attacks. These patients should also be counselled as regards the symptoms of a closed angle attack and the appropriate action to be taken if this occurs out of office hours. IOPs of over 50 mmHg are unlikely to respond to cholinergic agonists and should be referred immediately to an emergency ophthalmological unit.

Recommended anti-hypertensive/miotic agents. Pilocarpine is normally the drug of choice for both routine reversal of anti-muscarinic mydriasis and the emergency optometric treatment of subacute or acute closed angle attacks, whatever the cause. For emergency treatment of closed angle glaucoma use Gt. 2% for light irides and Gt. 4% for brown irides, every 5 min until the IOP begins to reduce, up to a maximum of 30 min. Quite substantial reductions in IOP (perhaps 10 mmHg) are usually seen within the first 10–15 min of treatment. Most IOPs return to normal within 30-45 min of initiating treatment.

It is possible that subacute closed angle attacks caused by the more potent longer acting anti-muscarinics such as cyclopentolate (rather than tropicamide) can recur some hours after apparently successful treatment with pilocarpine. This is usually due to the pupil re-dilating as a result of the different time course of action of the two drugs. Pharmacological acute or subacute attacks are usually caused initially by pupil block. This increases the pressure in the posterior chamber, followed by iris bombe and then angle closure. Because the crystalline lens of the pre-disposed eye is positioned more anteriorly than the normal eye, the risk of pupil block is greatest when the pupil is in the mid-dilated position, such as may occur in a re-dilating pupil in the above scenario. There may be some justification in these cases to consider treatment with physostigmine, which has a longer time scale (using a similar regimen to pilocarpine), to ensure that re-dilation does not occur.

Adverse effects. All the cholinergic agonists share similar adverse effects, with the greatest occurrences from carbachol and physostigmine and the least with pilocarpine. These are lid twitches, ciliary spasm, conjunctival congestion, prolonged miosis and cholinergic effects on the gut. Effects are also greater with the higher concentrations.

Cycloplegic for the emergency treatment of uveitis

The current treatment of acute anterior uveitis and cylitis is normally a combination therapy of a cycloplegic (to immobilise the inflamed iris and/ or ciliary body) and a topical steroid to reduce the inflammation in the affected eye. The management of this condition is primarily ophthalmo-logical but emergency optometric treatment can be initiated if emergency care is unavailable and the diagnosis is unequivocal. Although optome-trists are restricted to the use of cycloplegics (steroids being unavailable to the optometrist) treating anterior uveitis and cyclitis solely with a cyclo-plegic can be very effective. Indeed, some ophthalmologists have voiced the opinion that there may be surprisingly little to be gained from adding a steroid (certainly in mild cases) since the greatest therapeutic effect is probably attributable to the cycloplegia. Details of cycloplegic drugs can be found in the section on diagnostic drugs (Chapter 5).

Before initiating treatment, it is vital that the presence of any posterior synechiae is detected, since this determines the mode of emergency treat-ment; 360° of synechiae is likely to lead to pupil block and therefore intensive pupil dilation should be attempted. Several instillations of 1% cyclopentolate and 10% phenylephrine should be carried out with a view to breaking the synechiae. If no synechiae are present or they have been broken, the patient can be put on Gt. homatropine 2% t.i.d. or Gt. cyclo-pentolate 1% t.i.d. and referred for immediate ophthalmological care. Although the underlying cause of a single episode of unilateral acute anterior uveitis/cylitis rarely needs to be investigated, bilaterality or a recurrence needs urgent follow-up since there is likely to be some systemic cause. It goes without saying that these facts should be explained to the patient.

It should be noted that the treatment of posterior uveitis should be undertaken by an ophthalmologist because of its immediate sight-threa-tening nature and should be referred without further delay.

Suggested pharmaceuticals for optometrist's drug cabinet

Given the choice between multi-dose droppers and unit dose containers, the former may be the less expensive option. Clearly, this is dependent on the frequency of use.

Diagnostic drugs

Benoxinate hydrochloride 0.4% – Minims (Chauvin) or Ophthaine (Squibb) 15 ml bottles.
Tropicamide hydrochloride (PoM) 0.5% and 1.0% - Minims or Mydriacyl (Alcon) 5 ml bottles.
Minims phenylephrine hydrochloride 2.5%.
Cyclopentolate (PoM) 0.5% and 1.0%, Minims or Mydrilate (Boehinger Ingelheim) 5 ml bottles.
Florets 1 mg/strip (Chauvin).
Minims Rose Bengal 1.0%.
Aerosol saline (Bausch and Lomb) 360 ml can.

Prophylactic/therapeutic drugs for use in the practice

Given the relatively low use of these drugs, it is probably most cost effective to use the cheaper tube/bottle versions than Minims and replace them once they are used. Alternatively, if you have several practices, a box of Minims could be shared between them.

Brolene (Rhone–Poulenc Rorer) 5 g tube.
Emergency eye wash (Optrex) 500 ml bottle.
Chloramphenicol (PoM) eye ointment 1.0% (generic) 4 g tube.
Chloramphenicol (PoM) eye drops 0.5% (generic) 10 ml bottle.
Sno Pilo (Chauvin) 10 ml bottles 2.0% and 4.0%.
Viscotears (Ciba Vision) 10 g tube (gel).
Lid Care (Ciba Vision).
Otrovine–Antistin (Ciba) 10 ml bottles.
Opticrom allergy eye drops 5 ml bottles.

Further reading

Bartlett, J.D. and Jaanus, S.D. (1995). *Clinical Ocular Pharmacology*, 3rd edn. Butterworth–Heinemann, Oxford, UK
Doughty, M.J. (1996). *Drugs, Medications and the Eye*. Smawcastellane Information Services
The College of Optometrists Formulary (1994). Published by the College of Optometrists, 10 Knaresborough Place, London, UK

Superficial conjunctival and corneal foreign body removal

Background

Conjunctival and corneal foreign bodies are a common cause of emergency visits to the optometrist. Patients have varying degrees of pain or foreign body sensation, lacrimation, blurred vision, injection, and photophobia. A thorough and accurate history is critical and usually reveals a specific incident when the foreign matter entered the eye. Explicit details of the type of activity the patient was performing, the expected material of the foreign body, and the speed of the projectile must be determined. If the patient was hammering metal on metal or using a grinding wheel or drill, you must rule out the possibility of a penetrating injury. You must also be aware of other risks such as fungal infection with vegetative material injury, and pseudomonal infection in contact lens wearers. Lid eversion (and occasionally double lid eversion) must be performed to ensure that there are no further particles under the lid. Corneal foreign bodies (other than high speed) rarely penetrate the resilient Bowman's membrane.

Recommended tests

Slit lamp evaluation of the anterior segment to localise foreign bodies with topical anaesthesia. Instruments/methods of choice for conjunctival foreign bodies are ocular lavage with sterile saline, or removal of foreign bodies with surgical spears, forceps, foreign body spuds, or needles (Figure 6.1). Instruments of choice for corneal foreign bodies are sterile surgical spears or needles (usually 23 or 25 guage), and foreign body spud(s). An Alger brush is used to remove rust rings (Figure 6.1).

Rationale

Various instruments may be used by the clinician to facilitate removal depending on the location and depth of the foreign material. Multiple conjunctival foreign bodies may be removed by ocular lavage or irrigation with sterile saline. This method may be useful only for multiple foreign bodies that are not embedded and may in fact cause them to move around and potentially lodge elsewhere. Preferred to this is individual removal of each particle with a sterile surgical spear or sponge, which attracts fluid and foreign bodies by capillary attraction. Other options include using sterile jeweller's forceps to grasp the foreign bodies or using a foreign body spud or sterile needle to flick them out.

Corneal foreign bodies require more care due to the potential for scarring and possible but unlikely penetration of the cornea. Lavage is not generally successful at removing corneal foreign bodies as they are generally more embedded. The surgical spear and needle are commonly used as they are sterile and disposable. The surgical spear can be used as per conjunctival foreign bodies to attract and adhere the foreign body to it. This method is useful if you feel the patient may not sit still in the slit lamp. The spear is large, however, and inappropriate use can cause further abrasion to the cornea. Many practitioners use a needle or foreign body spud. Needles are sterile, disposable, and accurate in getting up under the particle and flicking it forward or scooping it off the surface. Needles come in different lengths and guages. The useful

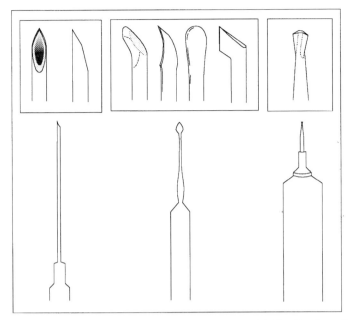

Figure 6.1 Foreign body removal instruments (not to scale) Needles (usually 20, 23 or 25 guage), foreign body spuds (golf club spud, foreign body spud, Davis or Ellis spud, Francis spud), and Alger brush (0.5 mm burr).

sizes are $\frac{5}{8}$ inch from 27 (small) to 20 (larger) guage. Care must be taken not to disrupt the basement membrane, but fortunately this is rarely a problem especially with good patient cooperation. Many practitioners prefer using foreign body spuds as they feel the blunt edges are less likely to cause corneal penetration. Many types are available with slightly different heads, e.g. golf club spud, needle-like spud and scoop-like spuds. Disposable foreign body spuds are also available. Both needles and spuds are used to get underneath the particle and flick or scoop it off the surface.

An Alger brush is used to remove stained epithelial cells from metallic foreign bodies. It is a battery operated instrument with a very small (0.5 mm or 1 mm) ophthalmic burr. This instrument allows the most accurate removal of the rust with the least adjacent tissue disruption. The Alger brush cannot 'drill' through the cornea as it has a mechanism that stops the rotating action of the burr when it encounters a certain amount of resistance. Bowman's membrane supplies sufficient resistance to stop the burr. The bevel of a needle or foreign body spud may also be used to remove rust stains.

A nylon loop is rarely used as it is generally ineffective at removing all except the most superficial foreign bodies. It may be considered by clinicians uncomfortable with sharper instruments.

Procedure

1. Take a detailed history of the patient's activities at the time the foreign matter got into the eye. The history should also include details of prior poor vision (e.g. of amblyopia), previous trauma or surgery, and family history of eye disease if possible.

2. Visual acuity must be measured before examination or administration of any treatment. Pupils and extra-ocular muscle function should be assessed.

3. Explain what you will be doing and that cooperation and good fixation are necessary to remove the foreign body. Obtain informed consent for these procedures. Topical anaesthesia may be considered if patient examination is impossible due to severe pain and/or photophobia. It is advisable to instil the anaesthetic after taking the visual acuity measurement if possible. (Make sure the anaesthetic is not within arm's reach of the patient as many have been known to take the bottle home with them to relieve the pain. Chronic anaesthetic abuse causes serious complications.)

4. Examine the anterior segment with the slit lamp. The cornea, conjunctiva and lids must be examined carefully, as should the lens, iris, and anterior chamber. The location of the foreign body and the depth of penetration must be accurately recorded (use an optic section). Foreign bodies on the visual axis must be evaluated carefully and the benefits and risks of removal discussed with the patient. Ensure the patient understands that scarring and vision loss may occur or may have already occurred due to the location and depth of the foreign body. Note the presence of epithelial and/or stromal oedema. Vertical tracking on the cornea suggests that there is likely to be an embedded foreign body under the upper lid. If lid eversion does not expose a foreign body, double eversion with irrigation should be attempted. Deeply embedded foreign bodies on the optical axis and penetrating injuries warrant referral.

5. Assess the anterior chamber with high magnification and a wide angle of the illumination source. Fully darken the room and dark adapt for a few minutes. Assess the anterior chamber for signs of inflammation (anterior uveitis) secondary to the trauma. Cells (white blood cells) can be detected with a shortened beam directed into the pupil and appear as fine white specks in the aqueous humour. Usually cells can be seen to follow the convection currents of the anterior chamber; upward posteriorly at the warm iris and downward anteriorly at the cooler cornea. The detection of flare (protein leakage) can be facilitated with a shorter conical beam which allows the normally optically empty anterior chamber aqueous to be observed. The observation of the anterior chamber for flare must be performed prior to the instillation of sodium fluorescein, as leaking of fluorescein into the aqueous could produce a false positive result.

6. Instil sodium fluorescein from a sterile strip moistened with sterile saline. Have the patient blink a number of times, then evaluate the surfaces with cobalt blue light. Observation of the fluorescence is enhanced by using a yellow filter (Wratten 12) over the observation system of the slit lamp. Consider everting the lid again as fluorescein will enhance the detection of a foreign body in the conjunctiva as well.

If a penetrating wound is suspected by history of grinding, drilling, or hammering metal, perform a Seidel test. Various sources describe this test differently. One option is to observe the wound site after fluorescein has been instilled into the conjuctival sac and is present uniformly in the tears. If aqueous is leaking, a clear stream may be noted coming from the wound site with or without slight pressure applied to the globe. The second and more specific method is to use one or two slightly moistened fluorescein strips to 'paint' the wound site. Relative hypofluorescence should be noted with the high concentration of fluorescein compared to the tears. Gentle pressure on the globe will reveal a green stream from the wound as the emerging aqueous picks up the fluorescein and fluoresces in cobalt blue light. It should be noted that high speed hot projectile foreign bodies may penetrate the cornea, iris, and even lens and leave very little evidence in the anterior segment. The iris, for example, will often 'seal' behind these particles, making it difficult to discern the entry wound.

7. Document the foreign body along with the area of any abraded epithelium or oedema in a detailed drawing.

8. Anaesthetise both eyes with one drop of topical anaesthetic (if not already done). Anaesthetising the fellow eye will assist with fixation and inhibit the contralateral blink reflex. Position the patient comfortably at the slit lamp and give the patient a fixation target for the fellow eye. Reinforce the need to keep the forehead firmly pressed against the headrest. Set the magnification to a moderate level (not high) and the illumination to a parallelepiped beam at an appropriate angle. Choose an instrument to remove the foreign body (bodies) depending on the location and depth of the material (see Rationale above). Secure the lids (an assistant or a lid speculum are rarely needed). Stabilise the arm of the instrument-holding hand. Introduce the instrument safely into the light of the slit lamp then move into the oculars. Remove the foreign body (Figure 6.2).

9. Reassess the cornea. Make sure the dislodged foreign body did not fall into the conjunctival sac.

(a) 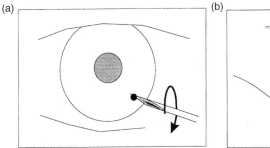 (b)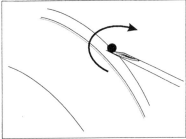

Figure 6.2 Removal of a foreign body using a scooping motion and a needle. The foreign body is flicked away from the optical axis. (a) Front view (b) magnified view of needle removing foreign body from epithelium.

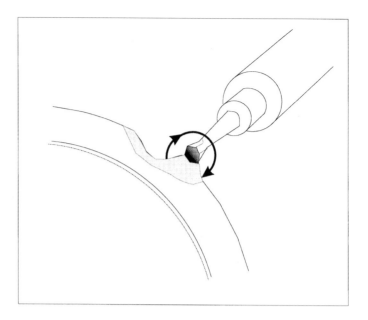

Figure 6.3 Alger brush removing a rust ring from the corneal epithelium.

10. Use an Alger brush to remove any rust ring (staining of the epithelium caused by oxidisation of a metallic foreign body). Choose the 0.5 mm ophthalmic burr. Rotate the tip to start the burr spinning. Advise the patient of the 'whirring' sound of the instrument. Hold the Alger brush tangentially to the globe and touch the burr to the stained epithelial cells until they are removed (Figure 6.3). Do not apply excessive pressure to Bowman's membrane.

11. Document carefully the extent of the abraded epithelium.

12. Take an intraocular pressure by applanation if possible. Low intraocular pressure could be indicative of penetration. Mildly low intraocular pressure may be incidental or indicative of a moderate anterior uveitis.

13. Dilate/cycloplege the eye. Evaluate the posterior pole with indirect fundus biomicroscopy and retinal midperiphery and periphery with binocular indirect ophthalmoscopy.

14. Consider pressure patching with an antiseptic (0.1% Brolene) or broad spectrum antibiotic ointment (0.5% or 1.0% chloramphenicol) if the patient is in extreme pain. Pressure patching is not recommended for injuries with vegetative matter or in contact lens wearers. Do not allow a patch to remain on the eye for more than 24 hours. Consider recommending analgesics for pain.

    Some practitioners do not advocate patching. Prescribe an antiseptic such as 0.1% Brolene or a broad spectrum antibiotic such as 0.5% chloramphenicol drops for those who are not patched. Choose an appropriate agent considering individual patient risks such as the *Pseudomonas* risk in contact lens wearers. Again, consider recommending analgesics for pain.

15. Book a follow-up appointment in 24 hours and instruct the patient on the importance of follow-up. Check for signs of infection and inflammation. If the epithelium is healed, consider discontinuing the antiseptic/antibiotic drops and starting aggressive lubrication. If corneal oedema remains, prescribe hyperosmotic ointment for night use and drops for day (if the patient can tolerate the stinging of the drops). If the epithelium is not healed, cycloplege again (depending on level of discomfort) and continue the antiseptic/antibiotic drops or consider re-patching the eye as above for another 24 hours.

Recording

Meticulously document the location, size, and depth of the foreign body and remaining abrasion after treatment. Monitor for resolution. Watch carefully for signs of infection, and unresolved inflammation and oedema, and alter treatment regimen accordingly. Monitor on subsequent visits for overlying epithelial erosion of the same area.

Interpretation

Most moderate corneal abrasions secondary to foreign bodies will heal in 1–2 days. Prolonged healing time may be noted in older patients and others with compromised corneal sensation, such as that induced by fifth nerve damage following stroke or chronic exposure.

Most common errors

1. Using the instruments inappropriately. A cotton-tipped applicator should not normally be used to remove conjunctival and especially corneal foreign bodies.
2. Inaccurately documenting the size/extent of foreign bodies and subsequent abrasion.
3. Failing to recognise the potential for intraocular penetration by poor history taking.
4. Failing to cycloplege the eye, resulting in significantly more discomfort.

Further reading

Clompus, R.J. (1991). Ocular foreign body removal. In *Clinical Procedures in Optometry* (J.B. Eskridge, J.F. Amos and J.D. Bartlett, eds) J.B. Lippincott, Philadelphia, Pennsylvania

Fingeret, M., Casser, L. and Woodcombe, H.T. (1990). *Atlas of Primary Eyecare Procedures*. Appleton and Lange, Norwalk, Connecticut

Messner, S.S. (1991). Corneal trauma. In *Clinical Optometric Pharmacology & Therapeutics* (B.E. Onofrey, ed.) Lippincott–Raven

Dilation and irrigation of the nasolacrimal system

Background

See Background in Lacrimal drainage evaluation section in Chapter 5. Dilation and irrigation of the nasolacrimal system is a useful test to determine if a patient complaining of tearing has a nasolacrimal system obstruction on the affected side. Stenosis of a portion of the system is common. Occlusion may occur from concretions secondary to fungal infection of the canaliculi. Tests such as the dye disappearance test and, more importantly, the Jones 1 test help to determine if irrigation of the system is indicated. Irrigation is performed when fluorescein dye instilled into the tear film spills over on to the face and no dye is recoverable in the nose. If fluid introduced into the canaliculi is noted by the patient in the throat, the nasolacrimal drainage system is patent. If more information is desired by the clinician with respect to the approximate location of the blockage, the effluent from the irrigation may be collected and the results analysed (Jones 2 test).

Recommended test

Rationale

Dilation and irrigation of the nasolacrimal system is the same procedure as the Jones 2 test with the exception being that in the Jones 2 test the effluent is collected and analysed. Many practitioners do not routinely collect the effluent as it makes the test more uncomfortable for the patient and the final result is not necessarily that useful. If the patient does seem to have a full or partial obstruction and the system is successfully irrigated, it may be assumed that the obstruction was either relieved by the irrigation or the blockage was partial. In any case, the patient may no longer experience tearing to the same extent as prior to irrigation and will be pleased with the results. If the tearing is not relieved by the irrigation and the patient requests further intervention, the practitioner may consider performing a Jones 2 test to determine the site of the obstruction.

Dilation and irrigation of the nasolacrimal system. Instruments: lacrimal dilators (long and medium tapers), lacrimal cannula (usually reinforced, 23 guage), 3, 5 or 10 cc syringe (10 preferred).

Procedure

1. Prepare the instruments. Attach a reinforced 23 gauge cannula to a 3, 5, or 10 cc syringe. Take the plunger out of the syringe and put a small amount of alcohol into the syringe, or alternatively place an alcohol pad into the syringe. Press the plunger and push the alcohol through the irrigating cannula to disinfect the inside of the instrument. Remove the alcohol pad. Disinfect all external surfaces of the instruments (cannula and dilators) with alcohol. Alternatively, the instruments may be autoclaved.
2. Fill the syringe with 2–3 cc sterile saline. Push some saline through the cannula to rinse the alcohol through.

Dilation

3. The patient should be fully informed of the risks and benefits of the procedure and give informed consent.
4. Recline the patient slightly in the chair. Use a magnifying lens (loupe) if necessary.
5. Anaesthetise both eyes with a topical anaesthetic in the inferior cul-de-sac.
6. Anaesthetise the superior and inferior puncta with a cotton tipped applicator soaked with anaesthetic. Have the patient open his or her

eyes. Pull the lids out of apposition with the globe and place the soaked pledget firmly on the inferior punctum. Have the patient close his or her eyes for several minutes such that both puncta come in contact with the applicator.

7. Pull the inferior lid away from the globe and place a dilator vertically into the inferior punctal opening. Use a dilator that will fit into the undilated punctum. This will almost always be the long tapered dilator.

8. Gently roll the dilator back and forth between your fingers.

9. Once the dilator is inserted 2 mm, turn the dilator nasally. Advance the dilator a little further while pulling laterally on the lid to straighten out the canaliculus. Continue to roll the dilator. Whitening of the punctal ring indicates expansion of the tissue. It is possible to note a snap of the punctal ring, but this is usually of no consequence. Do not force the dilator too deeply into the canaliculus. Do not force the dilator if resistance is encountered. The patient may feel some discomfort but should not feel any sharp pain.

10. If the punctum is not sufficiently enlarged, try again with the long tapered dilator and advance it further or introduce a medium tapered dilator immediately after the long taper.

11. Perform the primary dye test (Jones 1) after punctal dilation. If fluorescein is now recovered, the source of the poor drainage is likely stenosis of the punctum.

Irrigation

12. Direct the patient's gaze out and away from the canaliculus being irrigated. For example, have the patient look superior temporally to irrigate the inferior system.

13. Insert the cannula immediately after dilating. Pull the lid away from the globe and insert the cannula 2 mm vertically then pull the lid taut laterally to continue 1–4 mm into the horizontal canaliculus as with the dilator. The clinician may irrigate (introduce saline) at this point or consider advancing the canaliculus to the 'hard stop' position, indicating the cannula has come into contact with the nasal bone (Figure 6.4a). An appropriate hard stop indicates that all of the structures, including the canaliculus being irrigated, the common canaliculus and the valve of Rosenmuller, are patent. If the cannula meets with resistance, this is called 'soft stop' (Figure 6.4b). Obstruction or stenosis is inferred in the canaliculus being irrigated, the common canaliculus, or the valve of Rosenmuller, depending on how far in the soft stop is located. Do not advance the cannula if soft stop is detected.

14. Reach up with the thumb of the hand not holding the cannula/syringe. While watching that the cannula is not advanced further, apply pressure to the plunger to introduce approximately 0.5 cc of saline into the system. If resistance is encountered, withdraw the cannula and test that the cannula/syringe combination is not obstructed. Reintroduce the cannula.

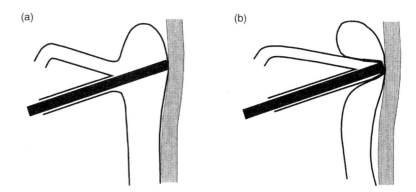

Figure 6.4 Diagrammatic representation of (a) 'hard stop' (b) 'soft stop' during dilation and irrigation of the nasolacrimal system.

15. The patient is asked to report when saline is felt in the throat. If saline regurgitates from the canaliculus being irrigated, it is likely that this canaliculus is obstructed or stenosed. If saline regurgitates from the contravertical punctum, have an assistant hold a sterile cotton tipped applicator firmly on that punctum and try to irrigate again.
16. Carefully withdraw the cannula. Keep talking to the patient to make sure that he or she does not move forward before the cannula is withdrawn.
17. (Optional: Jones 2) Have the patient lean forward and expectorate into a basin or blow into a tissue in order to recover some of the saline solution. Examine the basin/tissue with a Burton lamp or other cobalt blue light source for fluorescein.
18. Offer the patient a mint or lozenge as the saline may have an unpleasant taste.

Recording

1. The result indicates an obstruction if the patient does not taste salt or feel the solution in the throat.
2. Describe any regurgitation of saline. That is, regurgitation from the same canaliculus, indicating ipsivertical obstruction/stenosis, or regurgitation from the contravertical canaliculus indicating obstruction at the common canaliculus or farther.
3. After the patient has expectorated into the basin or blown into a tissue, record the presence or absence of fluorescein.

Interpretation

Normally fluid should exit from the system and be noted by the patient in the throat. A blocked system will offer resistance to fluid injection or cause regurgitation from the contravertical punctum. No fluid flow in the throat indicates a complete obstruction. Fluid noted in the throat indicates that the obstruction was relieved or there was a partial obstruction or stenosis. (See Lacrimal drainage evaluation: Jones 2 test interpretation in Chapter 5.)

Most common errors

See Most common errors (Jones tests) section in Lacrimal drainage evaluation (Chapter 5).

1. Not introducing the cannula quickly enough such that the punctum closes down after dilation.
2. Failing to respect the anatomy of the canaliculi with the cannula during dilation or irrigation, leading to patient discomfort.
3. Failing to use sufficient anaesthetic to achieve deep anaesthesia of the punctum in susceptible individuals prior to dilation and irrigation, leading to patient discomfort.

Further reading

Semes, L.P. (1991). Nasolacrimal testing. In *Clinical Optometric Pharmacology and Therapeutics* (B.E. Onofrey, ed.) J.B. Lippincott, Philadelphia, Pennsylvania
Semes, L.P. (1991). Lacrimal system evaluation. In *Clinical Procedures in Optometry* (J.B. Eskridge, J.F. Amos and J.D. Bartlett, eds) J.B. Lippincott, Philadelphia, Pennsylvania

Punctal and canalicular occlusion

Background

Dry eye and exposure keratitis are the most common ocular surface diseases encountered in optometric practice. Management includes the use of aggressive lubricants and lacrimal occlusion. Occlusion of the lacrimal canaliculi allows the reduced volume of tears to be preserved to better lubricate the ocular surface so that comfort is improved and the risk of serious complications reduced. Lacrimal occlusion is also useful for the marginal dry eye patient who wishes to continue wearing contact lenses.

Recommended procedure

Punctal occlusion; dissolvable intracanalicular collagen implants followed by evaluation and consideration for (semi-)permanent silicone plugs.

Rationale
Silicone plugs (punctal or canalicular) are expensive and reversal of the occlusion may be difficult in some cases if excess tearing or complications occur. Therefore, a diagnostic test is performed with dissolvable collagen implants in the superior and inferior

canaliculi. Collagen plugs dissolve in 4–7 days, at which time the patient is asked to return. Basal Schirmer testing and fluorescein and Rose Bengal staining before and after the insertion of the collagen plugs and observation of the tear meniscus height help to confirm any improvement to the tear volume and the likelihood of success. A diary of the patient's ocular surface symptoms is also helpful in determining if permanent plugs will likely be favourable. More than one trial of collagen implants may be needed to prove to the clinician and patient that permanent plugs will be a useful therapeutic option for their particular case. Patients with poor corneal sensitivity from nerve damage or chronic ocular surface disease often cannot notice an improvement in comfort, so the objective signs are more helpful. In these cases, repeated trials must be considered to monitor the corneal health to determine if occlusion is advisable. The patient should be aware that occlusion of the lacrimal drainage system usually will not eliminate the need for topical lubricants but may reduce the frequency of instillation.

Collagen plugs are available in varying lengths and 0.2 to 0.6 mm widths. Each sterile packet contains six plugs. Some practitioners cut dissolvable suture material to the appropriate length and use this in place of collagen plugs. Silicone plugs are available in two types: punctum plugs by companies such as Eaglevision (Tapered Shaft plugs), Labtician (FCI plugs) or Oasis (Soft Plug), and intracanalicular plugs by Lacrimedics (Herrick plugs). All silicone plugs are available in packages of two implants.

Dissolvable intracanalicular collagen implants

Procedure
1. Evaluate the patient carefully for dry eye and other ocular surface disease. Appropriate history should be taken including the specifics of the patient's current ocular surface treatments. Lid apposition and blink should be observed for abnormalities. Tear prism or meniscus, specular reflection of the tears, tear break-up time, fluorescein staining, Rose Bengal staining, basal Schirmer test, and other tests deemed appropriate should be performed. Side-effects of the therapy should be discussed and informed consent obtained. Allergy to (bovine) collagen and silicone should be investigated.
2. Prepare jeweller's forceps by disinfecting with alcohol. Alternatively, the instrument may be autoclaved.
3. Seat the patient comfortably at the slit lamp biomicroscope or in an examination chair capable of reclining. You can use either the slit lamp or a loupe for magnification.
4. Inspect the puncta and choose the largest implant size that seems likely to fit into the punctal opening without punctal dilation. The 0.40 mm size is the most commonly used.
5. Anaesthesia of the puncta and ocular surface is not recommended as it reduces the ability of the patient to detect an immediate improvement in ocular surface symptoms.
6. Grasp a single implant from the styrofoam packet (Figure 6.5a) either under the biomicroscope magnification or outside the slit lamp. The implant should be roughly perpendicular to the forceps tips.

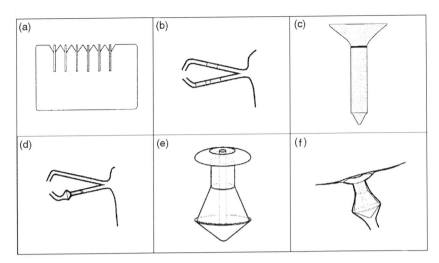

Figure 6.5 Diagrammatic representation of: (a) a set of six collagen plugs in their foam packaging; (b) hydrated collagen plugs in the canaliculi; (c) an intracanalicular (Herrick) silicone plug; (d) the flexible bell portion of the Herrick plug shown lodged in the canaliculus after collapsing when going through the punctal opening; (e) a punctal (Tapered Shaft) silicone plug and (f) a silicone punctum plug inserted into punctum. (Drawings are not to size.)

7. Instruct the patient to look upwards for the lower plug. Pull the lower lid away from the globe slightly to expose the punctum.

8. Place the implant partially into the opening vertically. Pull laterally on the lid to straighten out the canaliculus and advance the plug as far as it will go. Release the forceps. Close the tips of the forceps and gently push the rest of the implant into the opening while maintaining lateral positioning of the lid until it disappears beyond the punctal ring. If the implant does not go down below the punctal ring by this method, open the forceps and use the tip to push the implant all the way in.

9. Use two implants in the inferior and one in the superior canaliculus to effectively occlude the system for diagnostic purposes (Figure 6.5b). Occasionally single collagen implants may flush or reflux out of the system before they expand. Two to three implants in a canaliculus minimises the likelihood of the plugs refluxing out. This method also allows all six plugs in a card to be used.

10. Ask the patient to keep a diary of symptoms over the next 5–10 days, and arrange a follow-up appointment in 7–10 days. If symptoms and tear film evaluation suggest that permanent occlusion is appropriate, advise the patient of the benefits and risks of the procedure and obtain informed consent.

Recording. Record the type of plugs and the number of plugs inserted into each canaliculus. Record the results of any prior trial procedures. Using collagen implants, immediate improvement in symptoms or improvement in symptoms within the first few days is considered a positive response. It may take longer to note an improvement in any observable keratitis or conjunctivitis.

Interpretation. Carefully analyse and record patient symptoms and ocular surface signs including staining patterns and Schirmer test results. If a positive response is obtained with collagen plugs, semi-permanent (silicone) implants are generally inserted in the inferior punctum/canaliculus first. If occlusion is not sufficient to relieve symptoms to an acceptable level and ocular signs remain, the patient may require occlusion of the superior canaliculi. Before placing silicone implants in the superior system, perform a second diagnostic test in the superior canaliculus with collagen plugs. If this procedure is positive, insert silicone implants into the superior puncta or canaliculi. If epiphora is reported, do not proceed with superior occlusion.

Most common errors

1. Failure to use an adequate size or sufficient number of collagen implants to produce a positive response.
2. Inappropriately dilating the puncta, causing subsequent refluxing of the plugs out of the system before they can imbibe water and lodge in the canaliculi.

Silicone (semi-permanent) implants

Silicone implants may be considered after a favourable diagnostic test with collagen plugs. Options include intracanalicular or punctal type implants. In either case advise the patient of the risks and benefits of treatment and obtain informed consent

Advantages of intracanalicular (Herrick) plugs

1. Removal is accomplished by irrigation of the nasolacrimal system.
2. Insertion is much easier and does not require anaesthesia or dilation of the punctum.
3. The plugs are comfortable.

Disadvantages of intracanalicular plugs

1. Occasionally, the plug does not release automatically off the insertion stilette. This is easily remedied by using a foam applicator or sterile jeweller's forceps to detach the plug from the stilette in the sterile tray or while in the punctum. It can then be pushed down easily into the opening with the insertion stilette.
2. The possibility exists for the plug to become lodged and not able to flush through. Alternatively, the plug could flush through on its own and will be noted by the return of the patient's symptoms. In this case,

irrigation of the canaliculus should be performed before insertion of either another (larger size) intracanalicular plug or a punctum plug.

Advantages of punctal (tapered-shaft Freeman or FCI) plugs

1. Possibly more complete occlusion.
2. Low chance of the plug dislodging.
3. Plug is visible for monitoring.
4. Newer designs are more comfortable and hold in place better.
5. Tear flow can be controlled with certain plugs.

Disadvantages of punctal plugs

1. Deep anaesthesia is required as the plugs are resistant to insertion past the punctal ring. Insertion can be difficult and cause significant discomfort.
2. Equipment specific to the plug type is required to facilitate insertion.
3. Difficulty is often encountered in attempting to stabilise flaccid lids. The cotton-tipped applicator method is preferred in this case.
4. A long taper dilator may be needed first to dilate the punctum before using the attached or 1.2 mm dilator.
5. The implant dome rests above the punctal opening and can cause bulbar conjunctival irritation, especially with a concomitant entropion. This may be minimised with the tilted dome design of the FCI plug and with the softer dome of the Tapered-Shaft plugs.
6. Removal is possible but difficult as the wide area of the plug below the punctal ring must be pulled out.
7. Migration of the plug into the canaliculus has been reported with very small sized plugs or when the punctum has been excessively dilated. The plug then needs to be surgically removed. It is therefore important not to choose a plug that is too small.
8. Pyogenic granuloma formation has been reported.

Intracanalicular plugs. Herrick (Lacrimedics): these are available in 0.7 mm, 0.5 mm and 0.3 mm sizes. They are a golf tee shape with a soft collapsible bell (Figure 6.5c). The size designation is made at the narrow shaft.

1. Inspect the punctum. The 0.5 mm size should be chosen for all except the rare circumstances of very small puncta. The 0.7 mm may be considered for those patients in whom the 0.5 mm plugs have dislodged and flushed through.
2. Tear the lid off of the tray and remove the insertion stilette. Separate the two applicators and slide the foam along the guide wire closer to the plug.
3. Pull the lower lid down slightly and insert the plug approximately 60% of the way in until the collapsible bell rests on the punctum.
4. Direct the insertion stilette nasally while pulling laterally on the lid to straighten the horizontal canaliculus. Advance the plug into the canaliculus until it is out of sight (Figure 6.5d). Carefully remove the

stilette along the same line as the canaliculus. The plug should remain below the punctal ring.

5. Examine the punctum carefully. The plug should not be visible. If it is, use forceps or the stilette to push it down into the canaliculus a little more while pulling laterally on the lid.

If removal becomes necessary (epiphora or inflammation), irrigate the nasolacrimal system in the appropriate canaliculus (see Dilation and irrigation of the nasolacrimal system above). Successful irrigation confirms that the plug has dislodged.

Punctum plugs. Tapered-shaft Freeman plugs (Eaglevision), FCI (Labtician) and Soft Plug (Oasis).

The tapered-shaft type are available in mini size (0.5 × 1.3 mm length), petite (0.6 × 1.3 mm length), small (0.7 × 1.6 mm length), and medium (0.8 × 1.8 mm length) sizes. Each sterile packet contains two plugs preloaded on the dilation/insertion instrument. Tapered-shaft plugs are also available as punctum flow controllers, which are open through the centre of the plug, allowing some tears to drain.

The FCI variety have an angled dome to improve the anatomical fit above the punctum. The sizes available are: F3400 (standard 0.7 × 1.7 mm), F3800 ('umbrella' plug 0.7 × 1.7 mm), and F3100 (0.8 × 2.0 mm). Inserter/dilator instruments are required to insert these plugs.

1. Deeply anaesthetise the lacrimal punctum (and ocular surface) using the cotton pledget method (see Dilation and irrigation of the nasolacrimal system).
2. The small plug (Tapered-Shaft) is normally chosen first, but the appropriate size may be guaged with sizing tools (Eaglevision).
3. Recline the patient. A loupe is suggested for magnification.
4. Start with the inferior puncta after a positive diagnostic test with collagen plugs.
5. Immobilise and retract the lower lid by pulling down and laterally, or use a pair of cotton-tipped applicators, one on either side of the lid. Moisten the one against the conjunctiva with saline or anaesthetic.
6. Dilate the punctum with the dilation/insertion instrument or with a 1.2 mm dilator. Do not insert the dilator more than 2 mm into the punctal opening.
7. Immediately reverse the tool and insert the plug. Push the plug down to the level of the dome head.
8. Once in place, continue to hold the inserter in place and depress the release button.
9. Move the instrument away and examine the plug with the slit lamp.

If removal becomes necessary, grasp the plug with jeweller's forceps beneath the dome and pull from the punctal opening.

Recording. Record the type and size of plugs inserted into each canaliculus or punctum. Record the results of any prior trial procedures. Immediate improvement in symptoms, or improvement in symptoms within the first few days are considered a positive response. It may take longer to note an improvement in any observable keratitis.

Interpretation. If occlusion is not sufficient after inferior system occlusion, the patient may require occlusion of the superior puncta/canaliculi. Before placing silicone implants in the superior system, perform a second diagnostic test in the superior canaliculus with collagen plugs. If the response is positive and no epiphora is produced, silicone implants may be considered in the superior puncta or canaliculi.

Further reading

Barnard, N.A.S. (1996). Punctal and intracanalicular occlusion – a guide for the practitioner. *Ophthal & Physiol Opt*, **16**, S15–S22
Fingeret, M., Casser, L. and Woodcombe, H.T. (1990). *Atlas of Primary Eyecare Procedures*. Appleton and Lange, Norwalk, Connecticut

Index